A Yogi's Guide
to
Body Pride at Any Age

A Yogi's Guide
to
Body Pride at Any Age

by
Earl Ofari Hutchinson

**MID|DLE
PASS|AGE**
P R E S S

A Yogi's Guide to Body Pride at Any Age

Printed in the United States

Published by
Middle Passage Press
5517 Secrest Drive
Los Angeles, California 90043

Edited and indexed by Barbara Bramwell
Photographs by Angela Hoffman
Designed by Alan Bell

Publisher's Cataloging-In-Publication Data
(Prepared by The Donohue Group, Inc.)
Names: Hutchinson, Earl Ofari.
Title: A yogi's guide to body pride at any age / by Earl Ofari Hutchinson.
Description: [Los Angeles, California] : [Middle Passage Press], [2018] |
Includes bibliographical references and index.
Identifiers: ISBN 9781881032045
Subjects: LCSH: Older people—Health—and hygiene. | Body image. |
Exercise for older people. | Aging—Social aspects.
Classification: LCC RA564.8 .H88 2018 | DDC 613.0438—dc23

Library of Congress Control Number:
Middle Passage Press, Los Angeles, California

Table of Contents

A Yogi's Guide
to
Body Pride at Any Age

Introduction

The snickers, wisecracks, gasps, and raised eyebrows flew fast and furious in October 2017 when I published my first book on yoga, *A Skeptic's Guide to the Yoga Experience*. The less than complimentary reactions came from some family members, and some friends in person, and on my Facebook page. What prompted the outburst of unkind quips was the cover and the picture of me and my dress. Or, more particularly, my lack of dress. I went through a series of the more common yoga asanas in a *Speedo* brief.

Now what's interesting is there are hundreds of on-line photos of guys in Speedo bathing suits, or even in less, doing yoga poses and various other athletic poses. They are not all young Adonis's. Many are older guys who are bony, with guts, paunches, and wrinkles. However, they are all with no exception, white men.

So, for me, a 65-year-old plus man having the temerity to put his body on display, there were feigned gasps and comments, such as "Wow, you're being very risqué by showing your body." Or, "Please put some clothes on!" Then there were the chronic haters who live for the chance to hurl insults. In this case, I was their target. They slammed me with such invectives as, "namasgay," and that's "great porno stuff."

For many of those who took exception, and even offense at my brazen decision to literally bare my chest and body, this was too much. They refused to see the artistry, the physicality, the grace, and spiritual awareness, even adventure, that I brought to bear with the series of yoga asanas that I performed sans clothes.

The point of the book was not to showcase my body. It was to showcase my joyful discovery of yoga, and the benefit that it held for me. Yet, to some, this was completely lost. I was not offended by the crass putdowns. This was par for the course when it came to the display of one's body in America. Outside of the porn industry, the body building business, and maybe professional wrestling, showing the body in its natural state of undress is simply not something that most Americans can embrace, let alone revel in. Oh, ironically, there is one other exception, that's yoga. The hot (no pun) ticket item in yoga in 2018 was naked yoga. There are Facebook groups, studios, and videos that tout the merits of nude yoga.

The handful of negative comments made me think hard about why there is such a visceral, knee-jerk reaction to older men and women displaying their bodies, especially ones that they have worked hard to keep fit. I knew then I just had to confront this issue. And I'd confront that in a sequel to the yoga book. I'd take a hard look at the flash point controversies within the yoga, health, wellness, and even body building worlds.

A Yogi's Guide to Body Pride at Any Age takes that hard look at these issues. But it does more. It explores the issues of gender, race, religion, the social and cultural biases toward aging and physical exercise in relation to older men and women. These issues have been the subject of fierce debate. One issue in particular that has been especially prickly and garnered much atten-

tion in recent years has been the issue of body shaming especially in relation to seniors. *A Yogi's Guide to
Body Pride at Any Age* weighs in heavily on the side of
those who say no to body shaming, and yes to body
pride for seniors.

* * * * *

The reasons for the aversion to body displays are
well-known. The puritan tradition with all its hypocrisy and perils, that still hang heavy over much of
Western society is one reason. Another is the plague
of obesity which affects millions of Americans. This
causes many much shame, embarrassment, and guilt.
Many will do almost anything to avoid showing their
bodies.

Yet, another reason is the role religion has played
in drumming into millions that the body is a temple of
shame, rather than a temple of natural beauty. It must
be covered up at all costs. Despite decades of the loos-
ened faux sexual code of morality in the U.S. an un-
covered body is still seen as something to be scorned
and ashamed of rather than embraced and admired.

There were two other warning signs that there

would be a mild backlash to my revealing yoga poses. One was obvious. That is age. How many men aged 65 plus would dare strip down; as one of my acquaintances supportively said to me, to their skivvies and let it all hang out in a public display. She clearly saw my venture as a bold act of courage and daring on my part.

The other is less obvious, but no less revealing. That is race. I am not just a Senior, but an African-American senior. For many Blacks the puritan revulsion to nudity is deeply personal. The naked body implies loose morals, sexual licentiousness, and just plain immorality. That is certainly understandable given the long history of racial stereotyping of Blacks as sexually loose, and immoral. Nudity, or the barest covering, is not only taboo, it must be reviled and denounced, and in some religious circles preached against.

This has further instilled a collective self-consciousness in many Blacks about their bodies and sexuality. For them, they just simply can't give the detractors any more ammunition to slay them with. This more puritan-than-thou bias has cropped up on several occasion when issues such as gay marriage and abortion have been raging flash points of vitriol in America. Many conservative Black evangelicals have beat the drum louder than any other group against the alleged immorality of legalizing gay relations.

That's only part of the story of the negative reaction to my revealing yoga pictures. The other part is that many friends and supporters did praise my yoga book, and the pictures. They thought it was admirable that I embraced yoga and wrote a book about it. They were thrilled that I chose to showcase my body as a testament to the spiritual and physical benefits of yoga and wellness. My display of the raw, physicality of my body could not be separated from my yoga practice. Indeed, body pride is a crucial part of my journey into the yoga world and physical fitness.

* * * * *

When I began the practice of yoga in 2013, I did it with the hope that it would open up new vistas for me in my on-going quest to attain spiritual and physical wellness. There was more. Part of my quest was to confront the many myths and stereotypes propagated about older men and women and their inhibitions and reactions to them. The other part of the quest was to draw on my personal history and recount that history as a source of motivation and encouragement to more seniors to shed their fears about their bodies.

I'm certainly aware that the battle to change the mindset about wellness and the body is literally a matter of life and death for countless numbers of men, particularly Black men. The grim figures on illness, disease, and death are well known. HIV/AIDS, heart disease, diabetes, hypertension, asthma, stroke, prostate cancer, and of course, obesity has taken a heavy toll on Black men. They suffer more from chronic illnesses than any other demographic group in American society. This translates into the lowest life expectancy of any other group.

This is doubly compounded by two other troubling maladies. One is the lack of access to quality health care because of cost and the paucity of health facilities in poor Black communities. This is made worse by the often indifference of many doctors to African-American health needs. The other problem is denial. Many older Black men simply refuse to see a doctor when there are glaring signs that there is a medical problem.

The denial stems in part from the fear of hearing that they do have a major problem that requires long term, costly treatment and care. The psychological of trauma of this is too much to bear for many of these men, so they avoid a doctor's office like the plague.

The other part is suspicion. This is borne out of decades of mistreatment by, and hostility from, the medical establishment toward Black men. The memory of the brutal treatment of Black men in the infamous Tuskegee syphilis experiment on Black men for decades beginning in the 1930s hasn't been forgotten. There are other examples of this medical maltreatment toward Black men. The refusal of these men to closely monitor their health has frustrated many spouses and caregivers, and even many caring doctors.

I'm painfully aware that I could have easily been one of those fatal statistics, having battled obesity, a profound distaste of physical exercise, and anything remotely resembling paying attention to proper diet for many years. Fortunately, that changed. That change makes up a major part of my story in *A Yogi's Guide to Body Pride at Any Age*. The starting point begins in a time and place before I took pride in my body.

Chapter 1

From Fat to Fit

It was a typical warm and sunny Southern California autumn day in the mid-1970s. My nephew had pleaded with me that afternoon to take him over to a local park to shoot some hoops. Now, I hadn't touched a basketball in years, let alone played in a pick-up game. My idea of exercise was walking up a flight of stairs to the front door step of my house. He was persistent and really thought that I was capable of running up and down the court.

This was not a totally unreasonable assumption on his part. He knew that in high school I had been a highly touted high school football player and a champion shot putter on the track team. I had won many awards and accolades in both sports. In my more nostalgic moments, I still fancied myself as something of an athlete and hadn't totally lost my athletic prowess. So, it was a fairly easy call for me to say yes.

My fantasies of past athletic glory crashed hard after hitting the four-point mark in a two on two pickup game. I felt nauseous, and my stomach churned. I felt like vomiting. I staggered over to the grass and collapsed in almost a dead faint. The vomit that I felt coming, mercifully didn't get past my throat, but it was close. The sickness and dizziness I felt did. After what seemed like an eternity, I finally mustered enough energy to stumble to the car. I was 28 years old then.

For the next few days, my mind kept going back to that scene on the court. Why did that happen? Was I that out of shape? What could that mean for my long-term health prospects? It was not the first time that I had asked myself those tormenting questions.

In May 1973, I was part of a delegation of artists and writers who toured the People's Republic of China. The tour was fast-paced, and packed with many visits to communes, factories, theaters, and historic sites.

The one tour in particular that was the most memorable for more than just its historical and cultural value was the day I spent at the Great Wall.

The worst memory was that I couldn't make it up the first tier. I was winded and had to turn back and wait for the other delegation members to come back. What was even more galling I watched as several elderly Chinese couples walked just as casually and effortlessly up the various tiers of the wall.

Shortly after I returned from the trip, one afternoon my mother drove the nail home when she blurted out to me, "You're getting fat, look at your stomach." I weighed between 250 and 260 pounds. Her bluntness didn't offend me. It was another wake-up call about my body. However, neither this, nor the shortness of breath at the Great Wall, was enough to make me give up my one pleasure. That was eating, and not just eating, but eating whatever I could get my chops on.

One of my great delights was going to the old Van De Kamp Bakery near my house after classes at Los Angeles City College and grabbing a six pack of chocolate or maple glazed long johns. I'd wolf them down with a half-gallon of whole milk. My dinners were

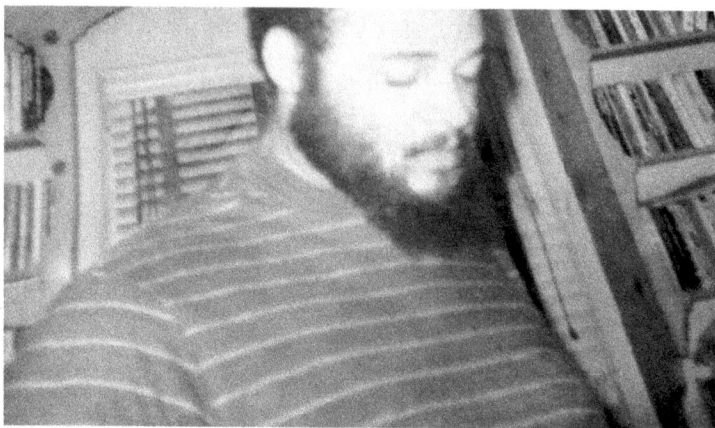

pork chops, fried chicken, meat loaf, ham, potatoes, greens, corn bread, and black-eyed peas, swimming in heavy oils. I usually finished dinner off with a slab of apple pie or chocolate cake. That was dinner. There were frequent snacks. They consisted of sandwiches, potato chips, cookies, and salted crackers. That went on well into the night.

I didn't even know then that you could fix foods any other way than fried. Baking, broiling or steaming poultry was a foreign concept to me. It was the old textbook Southern way of cooking and eating. My parents were as most Blacks back then, Southern folk. So, this was simply the way we as most Blacks in that era ate and continued to eat. The old habits didn't die hard, they didn't die at all.

* * * * *

So, what to do? It was not totally a newly found health epiphany that finally drove me to change. There was a good bit of vanity to it. I simply wanted to look, and yes feel, like an athlete again as I approached aged 30. So, I made three immediate changes. The first was I put myself on a regimen of no eating after 6 PM. I knew from the literature on diet that late night eating and snacking was a surefire way to gain weight. This was a major key to weight gain. There are volumes written on the physiological and biochemical dynamics of the body that make eating late-night meals, particularly junk food eating, detrimental.

The second change was to do a daily cleanse that consisted of drinking squeezed lemon or unfiltered apple juice every evening. I did this also to ensure that I stayed hydrated and to serve as a food filler substitute.

The third change was the most painful. I cut out the fatty stuff. I can't say that I went vegatarian. That would be a lie. I still liked my fried chicken. I discovered, though, that chicken could actually be baked and broiled, and still taste as good if not better. The trick was to vary my cuisine. A part of that was to add another food that I barely knew existed in my Rabelaisian eating days. That was fruits—apples, oranges, peaches, plums, bananas and nuts. They became staples replacing chips, cookies, and assorted sweets when I wanted to snack.

The key to making the changes work was exercise. I joined a summer pick-up basketball league. Twice a week I'd go to the gym or to one of the outdoor courts in the neighborhood. This rekindled the old sports enthusiast's desire in me. Even that wasn't enough, though. I wanted more. The more was something I never dreamed of. That was distance running. It happened almost by accident. A good friend at work one day asked if I wanted to do breakfast with him that Saturday.

The one catch was that he was going to enter a local 5K fun run, and we could do the breakfast afterwards. Almost as an afterthought, he asked, "Hey, why don't you come along and we can go from the race to the restaurant." I hesitated for a long moment, thinking what the heck am I going to do standing around at a fun run? I barely had any concept of what that event was. I reluctantly agreed. That Saturday he picked me up. When we arrived, I chatted with a couple of runners as he warmed up. I watched in pure fascination the throng of entrants—adults, kids, men and women of all ages, some even in wheel chairs. When the start gun sounded, the runners sprinted out. I then drifted over to the finish line to cheer my friend in.

I was struck by the joy on many of the runner's faces as they crossed the finish line. Despite their fatigue, they were exhilarated at their sense of accomplishment.

I wanted to have that same feeling of accomplishment. So, I started each morning with a walk and run of a few blocks. I gradually increased that to a mile, then two, then three. A couple of months later, I entered my first five K. It was a struggle to finish. When I did I was all smiles. I did it. I felt the same exhilaration. It was the runner's high.

* * * * *

Over the next few years, I ran dozens of local fun funs. I even traveled to other cites, and Rosarito Beach, Mexico to run races. My significant other, and soon to be wife, Barbara, also took up running. For the next two decades we were true running partners. Along the way, she won many awards at local races in various age categories. In time we even entered and ran 10 Ks, half marathons, and multiple marathons. We capped that by running the L.A. Marathon three times. We joined the mostly Black, Renaissance Runners Club in Los Angeles. It was a group of about 100 middle-aged Black men and women dedicated to running and fitness.

At aged 40 plus, I felt like I had become an athlete again. I even watched my diet more carefully. The biggest by-product of my new-found nirvana of athleticism, diet and exercise, was the weight loss. My weight now stayed steadily at 175 pounds. I added light weights to my regular five day a week workout routine. The experience of remaking myself at my age gave me almost a mystical feel of a transcendental new being.

What gave me the greatest satisfaction, however, was I had now turned 50 years old. This was an age when many older men, and that included many of my friends, were battling numerous health challenges. In almost all cases, an exercise regimen was a foreign concept to them. For me, though, there was no turning back. Even with the occasional injuries I suffered, which is an occupational hazard in the fitness business, I still managed to do something, a walk a sit-up, a stretch, something. It was not just physical. It was a mental and spiritual mindset that fueled my dedication to wellness and keeping my body and mind attuned to life and nature.

This all was a prelude, even warm-up, to yet another phase in my life's wellness journey. This phase would prove to be the greatest surprise of all. That was the discovery of the world of yoga. The title of my earlier book, *A Skeptics Journey Through the Yoga Experience,* best captured my thought about yoga. I had swallowed all the negative stuff about yoga. It was for women only. It was a New Age thing. It was for whites. Most of all, it was not something that an older man could do. The thought that yoga could be the pathway to a more complete mental, spiritual, and physically healthy lifestyle was totally remote to me. I was soon to be proven wrong.

Chapter 2

You Can Be a Warrior at Any Age

The image most of us have of a warrior is a young, muscular, supremely viral, kick butt action figure. That's in part the image rammed home through Hollywood's endless churning out of action and superhero movies. These movies are the staple of the Hollywood myth-making business. The notion that an older man or woman can be a superhero warrior figure is simply beyond laughable. However, Hollywood is not the real world. And it is especially not the world of yoga.

Let me digress for a moment about that in relation to yoga. I had a mental freeze frame for years of young, slender, athletic looking white women going through a variety of gymnastic looking poses, with barely pronounceable Hindu names. That would soon change. The change came by accident. I had just retired from my job as a loss control engineer at the California State Compensation Insurance Fund and I had time. So, I decided to take some classes at West Los Angeles College. One was a fitness class in the school's Kinesiology Department. The only class that was still open was yoga. With great reluctance, given my negative preconceived ideas about yoga, I enrolled in it.

The instructor and most of the students in the class were young women. This further deepened my initial doubts about taking the class. The instructor, though, was warm and extremely supportive and that did much to break the ice. The class quickly became an even greater eye-opener for me. My superficial, uninformed, and stereotypical view of yoga underwent a radical transformation. I quickly found there was more, much more, to yoga than those glamor, superficial commercial shots in magazines ads I had denigrated.

Yoga has a history, a very long and rich history. I vaguely knew that a huge part of that history was grounded in spiritualism and that its origin is in ancient India. This was only the start. To understand how yoga originated and its true purpose, I studied and read everything I could on it. One thing that stood out in my reading and study of the practice, was the central role of the warrior asanas. I was captivated by these particular yoga poses from the moment my instructor demonstrated them.

There are several basic warrior poses. Each one conveys strength determination, and even a tinge of ferocity. The poses, though, are the antithesis of the romanticized action hero concept, that being the take-no-prisoners, macho guy in popular culture. I learned there was a captivating story behind the warrior poses. The warrior posture or Sanskrit "Virabhadrasana" is a story of two ill-fated lovers in the ancient text. Their story encompasses the range of human emotions, love, hate, rage, violence, sadness, wrath, compassion, and forgiveness.

The warrior asanas all mirror the trials and tribulations, and the various aspects of the anguish of the

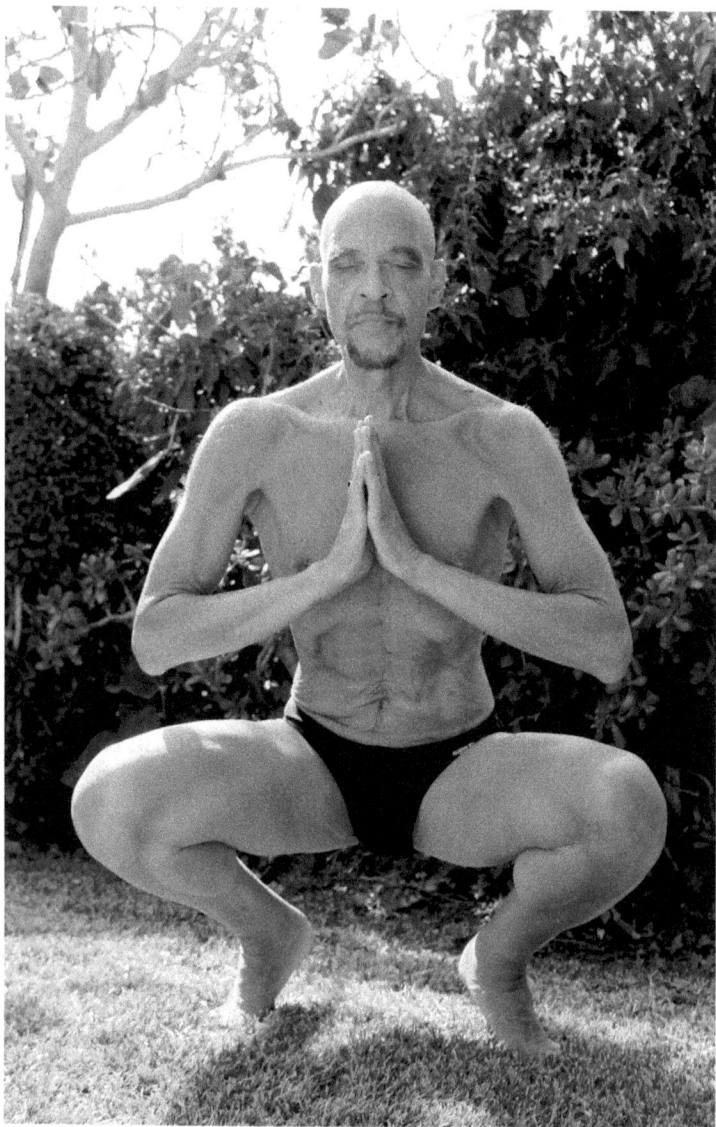

lovers. As with most tragic love stories, through the pain, suffering, heartbreak, there's a resolution. The male lover, Shiva, attains joy through the realization of his higher self. The higher self being the power to overcome tragedy and adversity by drawing on his inner strengths. The warrior in yoga is not a celebration or glorification of someone who wreaks destruction and mayhem or is endowed with super physical powers. He or she is one who is equipped mentally and physically to confront the various challenges that confront many in their daily lives.

*   *   *   *   *

What intrigued me each time I went through the three warrior poses was that anyone at any age who could stand upright could perform the warrior poses. In effect, they could be a warrior with practice and concentration. The poses are in reality a metaphor for life, the ups, downs, and twists, and ultimate triumphal pose in the asanas. For older men and women, they could have special significance given the many adversities and setbacks they often face in a long life. Each time I run through the varied warrior asanas at home and in my yoga classes, I think about the many challenges that I have faced. How I would sometimes sag under the burdens, then arise, straighten up, and continue my activities. The resilience, the gratitude and the humility, are depicted in the warrior poses.

The asanas instilled in me a keen awareness of the crucial connect between the body and mind. The warrior asanas, though, are more than just a physical and mental exercise. One posture is a back bend that is called the heart opener. This is an expression of openness, joy, and gratitude to life. It's a pose that demands the forgiveness of old grudges and old scores we accumulate over time against others for real or imagined wrongs against us. The heart opener serves to relieve inner tensions and release stress. The true warrior opens his heart to others in compassion and forgiveness. This is the ultimate test of strength.

The essence in finding the warrior in oneself is finding the capacity to let go of hurts, slights, and the tensions that result from holding on to bitterness, resentment, and animosity. This also helps to bring clarity and focus to problem solving. The strength, the mental and spiritual well-being, focus, and just plain determination to tackle a problem, dilemma or situation that seemed daunting, now become easier to attain.

* * * * *

While yoga proved a path to the discovery of the benign self in me, it's only one of many ways that older men and women can develop the same qualities. And let's be clear, one doesn't have to practice yoga to bring, clarity, strength and drive to their endeavors. The activities one can engage in for that are virtually unlimited; and can be found in sports, recreation, hobbies, and other favored pastimes. It just requires a willingness to engage the body and mind in an activity and stick to it.

One can think of someone who at one time or another had a sudden epiphany about their body. They took a gander in the mirror at their excess girth, or they suffered a physical malady. At that moment, they became instant converts to wellness. They quickly jumped into a taxing exercise program with the ferocity of a Marine drill sergeant.

After a short time, when you ask them if they

are still running, walking, playing tennis, handball, climbing, biking, or swimming, you get a shrug and a toss-up of the hands. Their gesture of resignation tells the whole story. The aura of defeat hangs heavy over them. There might even be a weak protest that this is only temporary, and that they'll be back at it again, soon. That's usually where it is left. Both know that the chances of that happening are slim to none. The promise to start up again at some vague, unspecified date, is as good as any.

*   *   *   *   *

I witnessed the withdrawal of many older men from the fitness ranks up close and in person in an aqua aerobics class that I enrolled in at a neighborhood Y in 2014. The weekly one-hour class was clearly designed for seniors. There were generally 15 to 20 participants in the class. They were all older women. Of those 15 to 20, I was almost always the only man. I say almost always because on occasion one or two men would show up for the class.

With few exceptions, it would be the first and last time that I would see them. Their drop-out became so predictable that some of the women from time to time would ask me how I felt being the only man in the class. I just shrugged, smiled, and went back to doing my front and back water kicks.

The Y had other classes on other days. At times there were more than a handful of men in those classes. However, this was the rare exception. It is tempting to chalk the absence of the guys in the exercise classes to squeamishness about being in a class with mostly women. Many men do attach a stigma to that. It's a huge disincentive for them to sign up and participate with any degree of regularity in these classes. They wrongly believe that these classes are for women only. The stark reality, though, was that coming to such a class, and putting the time and work in to get the benefit, took work and a commitment. Many men simply weren't willing to make the commitment.

It was easy for me to make that commitment because I had been a dedicated exercise devotee for thirty years plus my years in sports activity. This was just an extension of my overall commitment to the rigors of maintaining wellness. Yet, I did not judge or put down the men for not walking in my path. They'd have to unload a heavy train station full of baggage of negative conditioning and typecasting about what older men supposedly could and couldn't do with their aging bodies. They were victims of a culture that has erected powerful myths about aging. These myths have been unrelenting, and all-pervasive barriers to taking full ownership of their bodies and health.

There is one more dilemma. Older men are no different than younger men when they engage in an exercise program. They are competitive too. They will push themselves to outdo other men. They will push themselves even to outdo themselves. They'll push their physical limits sometimes to the breakpoint. For many older men, the mere thought of being outdone in a physical activity by a woman is too much to bear for the male ego. This shouldn't surprise. In Western society, men traditionally have been raised to look with scorn on anything that's perceived as "girly." The universal admonition and put down for many boys is, "You're acting like a girl." And boys that are perceived as less "masculine" catch hell from other boys.

Aggression and competitiveness are drilled into them early on and reinforced in small and large ways as part of society's social norms well into adolescence and adulthood. Numerous studies have shown that men are groomed to be more competitive than women.

For instance, in one experiment, researchers had male and female students work adding columns of two-digit numbers and paying them for their correct responses. They were then put in a tournament where only the fastest problem-solver got paid anything. Male students were far more likely to opt to compete in the tournament than women students. The researchers attributed the gender disparity to typical male over-confidence in their adding abilities and their intense desire for competition. The athletic arena is even more ferocious in bringing out the best and worst of the conditioned male response to competition in men.

So, it's no surprise that studies have found that over 50 percent of those who start an exercise pro-gram will drop out within the first six months. That figure is probably too low and the time frame for their dropping out is far too high. With older men that even presupposes that they'll start such a program in the first place. Age then is always the highest hurdle for many men and women to jump over. How could it be otherwise when they continually hear others say, "Hey you're too old for that."

Chapter 3

Hey, You're Too Old for That

About once a month I go to my chiropractor. This is the same chiropractor I have been going to for more than 20 years. I have heard the question from him so often that I can predict exactly when he'll ask it. In fact, I can recite it in my sleep verbatim because it never changes, "Are you still running?" The special emphasis is on the "you." At times, the question seems as if it's part indictment, part inquisition, and in greater part, amazement.

He was really saying why is someone your age still running several miles every day. On better days when I visit, he'll soften that with an admonition to run slower, pace yourself; and most importantly be sure to run on a soft surface. Then as part of his take care of your body admonition, he reminds me that I am just about the last man standing in the running club I mentioned earlier; the now defunct Renaissance Runners. By that he means, I, and maybe a couple of others, are the only one of the original club members who are still running.

He's right about that part at least. At its peak the club had nearly 100 members who ran regularly. They were all aged 45 plus. Over the years, the full complement of physical maladies took their toll. Hardly a month went by that I didn't get an email from the unofficial club chronicler about the hospitalization or death of one of the members.

I took due note of this. In nearly every case, the departed had been a close associate, friend, and in some cases active running or training partner. I had fond memories of the races that we entered. More times than not, they would almost always beat me to the finish line in one of the 5 Ks we raced. They were the epitome of senior athletes who took supreme care of their bodies and were in tip top shape. It was hard for me to imagine them transitioning or incapacitated. Yet, that was the bitter reality I had to accept

My chiropractor stood the question of my continuing to run on its head and reminded me that I was in some way special way almost a freak of nature. Here was a man my age who seemingly beat the odds and was still out there doing such an intense, vigorous workout as running. I didn't see it that way. I knew that there were other men my age and older who were devotees of physical fitness activities and who were in superior shape and in excellent health.

One, in particular, was a close friend. He was nearly age 80 and not only still running 5K road races, but winning medals in them. I'd often see him training during the week on the streets stripped to short running singlet and short running tights. I'd think wow, what a body! He, and men like him, were classic road warriors with no age qualifier tossed in. They proved it by their devotion and commitment to wellness. They rejected, as I did, the notion that an aging male body is a spent body; a body that had to be preserved like a stuffed specimen at the Smithsonian Museum.

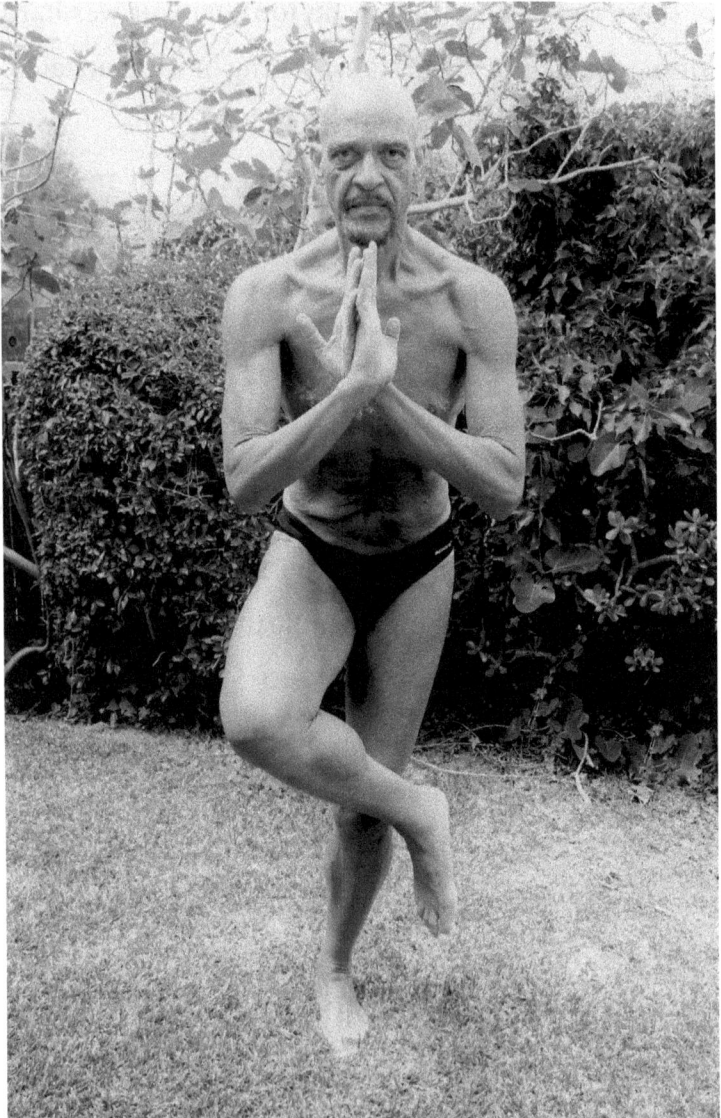

I couldn't be too harsh with my chiropractor. He was well-intentioned and truly concerned about my well-being. But I also knew that he was repeating the prevalent and deeply held myths and misconceptions about aging men and their health and bodies. The astounding thing about that was that the myths and misconceptions that underlay his question to me about my running have been thoroughly debunked in studies and by many researchers into sports fitness and its effect on older men and women. Here are the most common myths, misconceptions and warnings to those age 60 plus:

Myth 1
I'm too old to exercise

This is my favorite myth. It flies in the face of everything that we know about exercise and aging. Moving the body decreases, not increases, the risk of being hit by the big killers, heart disease, dementia, high blood pressure, and even cancer.

Myth 2
At my age, I need to rest and take it easy

This has all the earmarks of an old husband and wife's tale. I remember that in one series of interviews with older married men, several men said that they had given up sex because it would have an adverse effect on their health. It seemed laughable. Obviously, it wasn't to the men who believed that and worse practiced it. To debunk this, you don't have to cite the medical texts or studies. The answer is in the popular admonition "use it or lose it"

Myth 3
The danger of injury is too great

There's a kernel of truth to the injury risk in exercise. In fact, there has been much written on the subject of injury and older men. However, that risk is there for anyone at any age. Just ask world class athletes in track, football, basketball, tennis, and other sports. They are hardly geriatric, and they regularly suffer major injuries.

Injuries can and do happen when someone over

taxes weak or tired muscles, joints and ligaments Or, they are dehydrated, or have an illness, or prior injury that has been aggravated. Injuries are a common problem for some men in yoga. It's not the yoga that's the cause. It's the men overdoing it.

The watchwords are moderation, rest, and proper warm-up and stretching before a heavy-duty exercise workout. This applies to young as well as older women and men.

Myth 4
It's too late to start now

Every study that's ever been done on the benefits of exercise for older men shows that moderate exercise, be it walking, aquatics, tai chi, biking, light weight training, and of course, yoga, has tremendous cardiovascular and mental stimulus benefits. These exercises can even be done by someone who relies on a walker or even who's in a wheelchair. So, even a physical disability can't be hidden behind as an excuse to do nothing.

Myth 5

Your age determines your optimum
fitness routine

This is my second favorite one. It usually goes like this after you've told someone younger than you that you've started a fitness program. "Oh, that's great, but be careful don't overdo it at your age." The not so subtle message is that anything more strenuous than a game of tiddly winks will be extremely hazardous to your health.

Obviously, it's important to exercise caution with any physical activity. This rule holds true for anyone at any age. The American Academy of Orthopaedic Surgeons recommends that no matter what the intensity level of a person's workout, it should include aerobic, strengthening and flexibility components, as well as exercises that improve balance. However, there is no one size fits all type of fitness activity for any group of individuals at age 50 plus. It depends on many factors. The most important of which is the physical health of the individual and their mental approach to the activity.

Many senior competitors in track and swimming events say they are in far better shape than when they were 20 and 30 years younger. The age question has more often than not been a coy cover that many older persons use to convince themselves that they are too old to do anything that requires more effort than getting off the couch.

Myth 6
The baby boomers are the most physically fit generation ever

This is my third favorite myth. I've heard it said so often that I almost believe it. Maybe, a part of me wants to believe it because I'm one of them. Baby boomers, that's those who were born between 1946 and 1964, do have the media hype of being the most fitness-conscious, presumably because of their education, savvy, and higher income.

While there are a lot of over age 50 men biking, running, swimming, and in gyms and fitness centers, there are millions more who aren't. Only about one in five men and women in that age group do any kind of exercise on a regular basis. Sitting at a computer hour after hour hardly counts as an activity that poses a physical challenge. This is what many baby boomers do. Why? Because they still hold down full-time jobs, run businesses, and attend meetings. The pattern of inactivity often goes on into their leisure hours.

The truth is that as a group, baby boomers are in worse shape than their parents. West Virginia University researchers in March 2013, reported in the March 2013 issue of the *Journal of the American Medical Association,* they had a higher rate of poor health and disabilities than did their parents' generation. There's more. The Centers for Disease Control and Prevention has predicted a decline in life expectancy for many of that generation as obesity leads to an increased rate of hypertension, diabetes, high cholesterol, and chronic disease.

The image of active senior living makes good copy, but there's little truth to it. Yet, there could be, and at least the one in five seniors who are active, be it in one of the fitness and wellness regimens, including the one that's my passion, yoga, provide a solid model for others who do in fact want to be one of that one in five.

* * * * *

Each one of these, and other myths, misconceptions, and untruths, are major impediments to older men and women becoming wellness practitioners. On the other hand, each one of them is smashed every year at the National Senior Games. Tens of thousands of men and women take part in the games nationally. There are nearly two dozen events. The times for the participants in the events are as expected slower in most cases than for those in their 20s. But even that's relative. When statisticians factor in the age component gradation say in a 50-meter swim or 100-meter dash for the senior competitor, the numbers are remarkable.

Many of the age 50 and 60 plus men and women repeatedly insist that they are faster and stronger at their age than when they were 20 and even 30 years younger and competing. This is not hyperbole. They pay much more attention to their diet, and training. They bring a higher level of focus and consistency to their workouts than when they were in their 20s.

In the 5 K races that I ran in for more than two

decades after age 40, I noted that the times in the age categories from 50 to 60, 60 to 70, and even 70 to 80 for many men in those age categories were often faster than many of the top times in the younger age categories. There were some men 60 plus who actually competed in the younger age categories and more often than not earned a place.

One senior athlete who stands as the model for athletic prowess for older men is Don Pellman. At the San Diego Senior Olympics in 2015, the 100-year old Pellman drew national attention when he shattered the senior record in five events, the high jump, long jump, shot put, discus and 100-meter dash. They are hardly soft leisure time events. They require a high degree of training, skill, and determination.

Even more remarkable in some ways was that he had been a track specialist for many years yet had never suffered a major injury while racing or training. He attributed that to a lot of luck. This is undoubtedly true, but luck wouldn't have meant much, in fact almost certainly would have run out, without his close attention to rest, diet, and proper training. Admittedly, he was the rare specimen who could accomplish those feats. However, he proved once again that the barriers to being fit can be obliterated at just about any age.

There is one other myth that the older male competitors in the senior games exploded. That is the men who regularly competed were retired. And, they had lots of time on their hands, and could afford to put the time into training and conditioning their bodies for the competition. The majority of the men either worked full or part time jobs, or ran businesses, and had families.

They squeezed their training in between busy work schedules and their family responsibilities. For them it wasn't just their exceptional athletic ability, or a fierce, iron-willed determination. It was also time management. They figured out how to do the proverbial rendering unto Cesar (their jobs) and render unto the heavens their workout routines. The key was focus and discipline in every aspect of their training.

They did something else that running track and swimming required. They had to undress. Here were older men and women on the track and in the pool in singlets, shorts, and bathing suits. Their bodies were on display along with their athletic talents. These age 60, 70, 80, and 90-year-old men and women were peak age group athletic competitors and their bodies showed that. They took pride in getting their bodies to that point, and there was no shame in showing them. Unfortunately, far too many other Americans don't see anything of beauty in their body, but only shame.

That shame has coined its own term and controversy. The term is body shaming.

Chapter 4

Saying 'No' to Body Shaming

When I published my yoga book with the pictures of me doing the varied asanas in my *Speedo* bathing suit and then posted some of the pictures on two Facebook health and wellness sites, the reaction from some was swift, and even brutal. No matter how the critics worded their displeasure and even offense at the photos, it boiled down to, "Please, put some clothes on."

No matter how many pictures I showed of Indian yogis, who are the world's great yoga master's, in loincloths, or in scanty attire. Or, pointed out that yogi's had been doing and photographing themselves doing their asanas in bikini bathing suits since the 1970s, it made little difference. The response was still yes but put some clothes on! Now, I emphasize some were offended. Others weren't. They saw the artistry in the pictures. They admired the physical conditioning, and even daringness, that a near 70-year-old man could and would show in posting them.

I used their criticisms as a teaching moment. I continually hammered away that doing yoga undressed, or without being attired in trendy and expensive yoga wear, are not incompatible. Those who only saw the pictures as crass exhibitionism by an older man were aiding and abetting the silly, detrimental, and absurd phenomena that in recent years has gotten its own label. That is body shaming. This has long been a big point of debate, controversy and acrimony among many about those who display their bodies. Some don't like it if you're too fat. Some don't like it if you're too thin. Some don't like it if you're too short, tall, or possess a storehouse of other body traits not regarded as the norm of what conventional body beauty standards are supposed to conform too.

* * * * *

One person who knows a little something about body shaming because she has been a prime target of body putdowns for so many years, had this to say about it, "I realized that you really have to learn to accept who you are and love who you are. I'm really happy with my body type, and I'm really proud of it." Serena Williams should be. After all, she's heard the endless wisecracks and digs, "She's too big," "She's too muscular," "She looks like a man." Her monster success on the tennis court. Her wealth. Her success as an entrepreneur. And even her lashing out at them in open letters, and in public appearances, have done absolutely nothing to silence these detractors. If anything, it's made them even more emboldened to attack her body shape. This isn't all. Williams even expressed worry in a TV appearance in May 2018 that they'd even go after daughter.

The body shaming took on an even edgier, malicious tone as she approached middle-age. The reason: she was still winning championships and still beating women who were almost half her age. This is al-

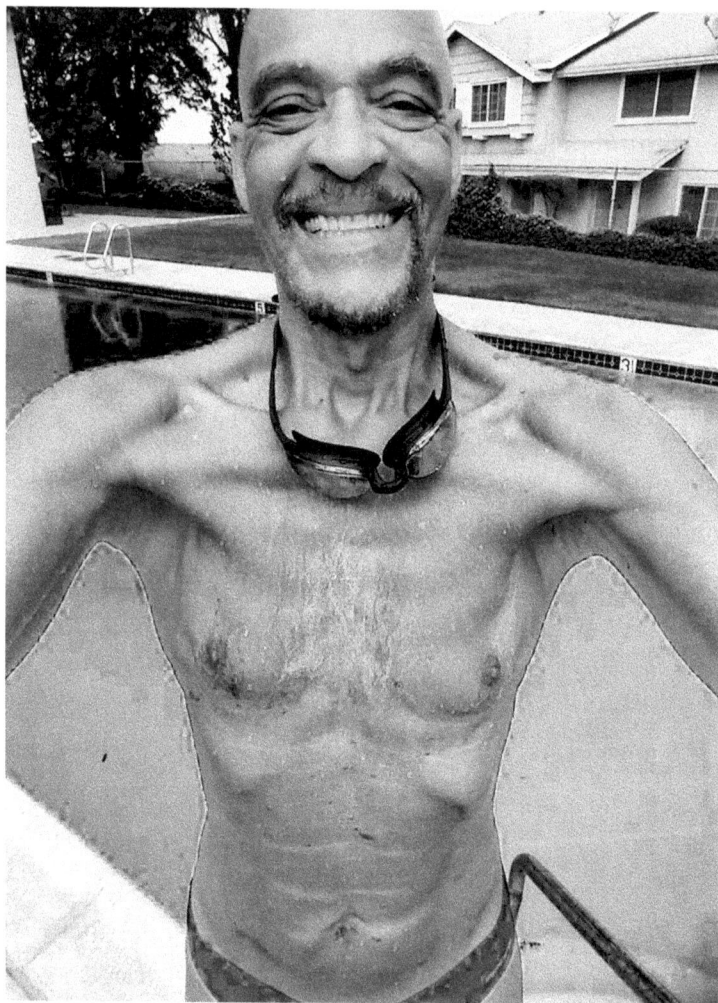

most sacrilege within and without the sports world for a middle-aged woman. Williams was undaunted. She had one more answer to the haters. She posed in a bold bikini and posted it on Instagram, while slamming and poking fun at the body shamers. She doubled down with a bare breasted picture of herself as a pregnant mother in June 2017, on the cover of *Vanity Fair* magazine.

The hateful reaction Williams got for decades can be repeated a thousand times, and a thousand different ways daily with anyone who has what's perceived to be an irregular body type. The hateful reaction to this bars many from putting their body on full unclothed or near unclothed display. This is mostly an American phobia. Most Europeans do not have this wrong-headed view of the human anatomy. There are nude beaches, nude festivals, and legions of nude societies in Western European countries. I'll talk more about this in my next chapter.

Even here, though, there is a hitch. The retort is that this is true about the Europeans and their liberal view of the body. However, the ones who are prancing around in the nude are all young persons. How many old women and men, they say, do you see running around at beaches with tiny bathing suits on or nude? The truth is that there are plenty of older persons who do. Like any other belief, no matter how erroneous, when bolstered by an unyielding puritanical moral code, that a naked, or scantily dressed body, equates with sin and immorality, it's a tough one to get around.

*   *   *   *   *

The roots of body shaming go deep. It encompasses a blend of religious beliefs, traditional family values, and the jaundiced conception of the role of women. There's also a hefty dose of self-loathing and guilt about one's own body. The Victorian ideal of body chastity ruled for decades in Western society. Women were considered harlots if they were not wrapped in a full regalia of corsets, brassieres, petticoats, hoops, and layers of dresses. For men, it was suits, ties, hats, and overcoats, even on the hottest summer days. In those times well-to-do men would not dare step out in public without a heavy layer of elegant clothing.

There's more. The more is the *Bible*. It is the cornerstone of Christian belief and practice. There are numerous passages in the *Bible* that decry nudity, and brand it as a shameful act and a sin. There's an irony in this since in one of the very first passages in Genesis that tells the story of Adam and Eve, it states, "And they were both naked, the man and his wife, and were not ashamed."—Genesis 2:25. However, after their flop into sin and their tumble from the Garden all rules about the body and nudity no longer applied. From then on clothes were the order of the day.

That doesn't end the Biblical story about clothes and the body. In several *Bible* passages, not only is nudity condoned but it is demanded by God. There's Job's nakedness in his humility toward God. There's David's nakedness in his worship of God. There's Isaiah's nakedness in preaching in the Word of God. The Isaiah story is especially tantalizing. Here's the exact passage, "At the same time spake the Lord by Isaiah the son of Amoz, saying, Go and loose the sackcloth from off thy loins, and put off thy shoe from thy foot. And he did so, walking naked and barefoot."—Isaiah 20:2.

Isaiah being the dutiful servant of God that he was he obeyed and preached naked as a sign to Egypt and upon Ethiopia that they would be conquered by Assyria and brought back naked and barefoot. The common thread in each of these passages is that it is not nakedness for nakedness sake. God had a specific purpose and task for them to accomplish to fulfill His preachments. Nudity was a part of that.

Fast forward two millennia after Christ's birth. More than one personality in America has discovered to their profound shock and sometimes embarrassment that they were the target of torrents of abuse. Why? Because they dared break convention and bare all, or more of their body than the public deemed appropriate. In almost every case, they were young women, or young gay men who displayed photos of themselves in varied stages of undress, or nudity. The nit picking quickly began about some part of their anatomy that was a turn off. They were young persons at least.

What happens when one who is not young goes bare? Then it's a scandal. But it doesn't have to be.

Chapter 5

Saying 'Yes' to Body Pride

The only older men who get a pass from the body shame police are those men who show their stuff in varied poses in body building contests. They can wear the skimpiest bikinis and as long as they're muscles shine and ripple, and they appear young, there are no shouts at them to put on some clothes.

Basketball great Kobe Bryant got a taste of body shaming when some months after he retired from the game he took a vacation with his family to Italy, a country where he spent his childhood years. While out and about a photographer took a shot of a shirt-less Bryant. This touched off a mini-uproar when it cropped up on Instagram. Bryant had visibly gained weight. He now no longer looked like the trim, physically imposing Bryant that basketball fans were accustomed to seeing.

There was a backlash. A horrified Bryant quickly deleted the photo from Instagram and replaced it with a photo of a black image captioned "Mamba mode #blackout." This was his moniker during his basketball glory days.

The athletically gifted Bryant was the target of the body shaming crowd, after he had the temerity to display his body *sans* shirt. Now, the man who is decades older and without the superstar athletic pedigree of a Bryant that bares his body would be the brunt of merciless criticism. There are harsh consequences for this rigid view.

The first is self-esteem. A man who is disdainful of others for the shape of their body—it's too fat, too thin, too small, too blemished, and so on—are more likely to find faults with prospective mates. And they are also more likely to have eating disorders. The body phobia doesn't just crop up when a man hits a certain older age. It can start early.

They fear that weight gain will mark them as the butt of ridicule. This fear pushes some men to grasp at anything to avoid the jibes. They punish themselves with starvation diets and frenetic exercising. They are suckers for fad nutritional supplements that make all kinds of phony, or at best, unproven claims to be the magic elixir to shed pounds and make a guy look like Charles Atlas virtually overnight.

The problem is doubly compounded when sex is tossed into the equation. Studies have confirmed that when men view the body solely as a sex object they are more likely to be hyper-critical and hyper-sensitive about uncovering their body. They fear that they will somehow come up short on the manliness scale since sex is still seen by many as the earmark of a man's virility. These men are also more likely to engage in body shaming of other men.

This has yet another dire consequence. Many men are put out that their bodies do not fit the idealized perception of the body beautiful mirage pumped by Hollywood and the media in countless advertisements for

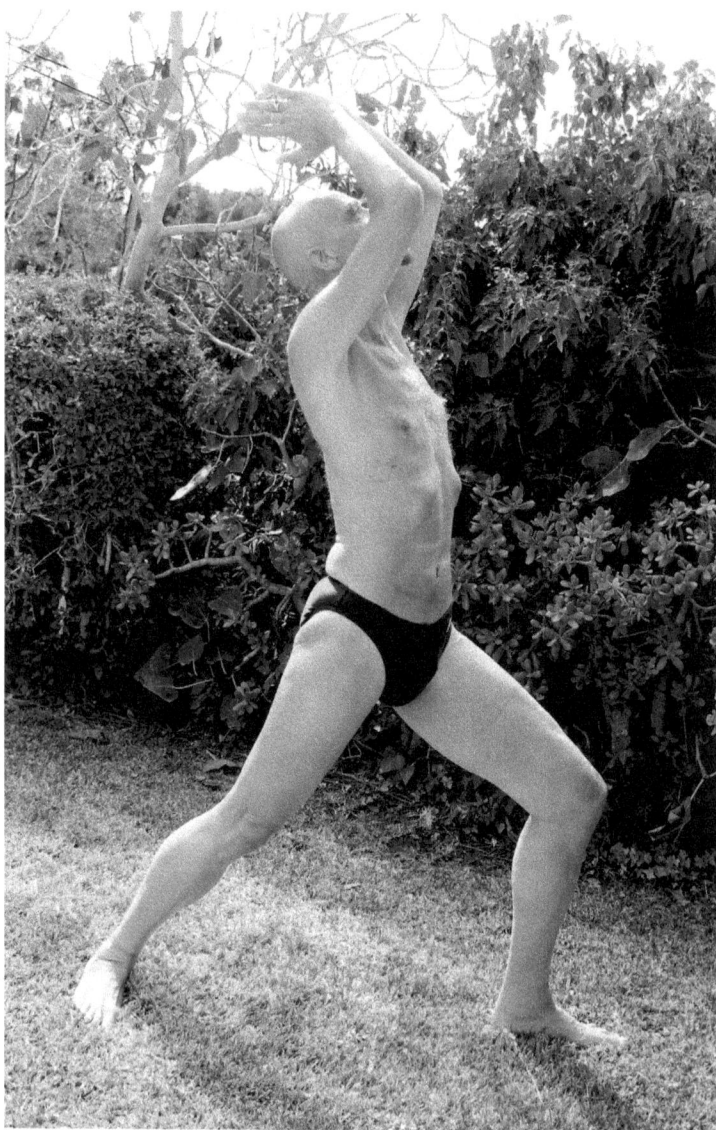

products. As a result, they are more prone to suffer bouts of depression and binge on alcohol and drugs. They are also more likely to seek counseling and treatment.

How great then is the body shaming problem? It's pretty great. Studies compiled by researchers at Bradley University in 2013 found that a whopping "95% of college age men are dissatisfied with their bodies on some level. The study found that American men, and probably men in other countries, feel under intense pressure to look like the touted body masculine beautiful image. They sought to pump up their bodies, or slim down in an effort to be both lean, and at the same time add bulk to their muscles. The gargantuan number of college men who expressed dissatisfaction with their bodies were no different than the number of men in general who also felt the same way about their bodies.

Another study found that over 90% of men struggle in some way with body dissatisfaction and with the negative affect (negative opinions of self), and negative emotions and thoughts about their bodies. Unlike women, though, men are more prone to suffer in silence, since it is still considered unmanly or weak for men to express their personal anguish to others, especially other men.

* * * * *

Much less is known and has been written about the effect of body shaming on older men. In fact, I couldn't find one article on this subject after an extensive Google search. There are many articles on medical websites and in men's health magazines and publications that cover a range of health issues. But I found nothing that specifically addressed the fears and phobias of aging men in relation to body imagery.

From what I glean from the shop talk when older men get together is that much of the chatter and focus is on the body shapes and sizes of women. This is heavily tinged with talk of sex. One tip-off, though, about the depth of body phobia among older men, particularly Black men, is the almost total absence of any pictures of older African-American men in anything less than full dress regalia on Black oriented health and wellness groups on Facebook.

One explanation for the body phobia among Black men is the long-standing racist sexual fantasies of Black men and their bodies, particularly their sex organs. They have been the prime target of the litany of negative stereotypes and negative typecasting of them as sexual super studs always on the prowl (usually for white women). This has instilled a cultural and racial conditioned extreme hyper-sensitivity among many Black men about putting any part of their body on public display.

*   *   *   *   *

There is yet another ugly consequence and reason for the heightened guardedness by Black men about their bodies. A 2017 American Psychological Association study found that even though American born white and Black men are roughly the same height and weight, the perception is that Black men are bigger and stronger, and more physically muscular than white males. This false notion strikes to the heart of the old stereotype of the physically dominant and thus menacing Black buck. It is only a short step from this false perception to justify the sort of mayhem from lynching in decades past to police over use of deadly force perpetrated on Black males.

It's no surprise then that proper dress is a paramount measure of dignity and class and pride for many older men. Anything less, is considered a violation of the code of how men, of all ages should display their bodies. This inflated, and culturally induced compelled modesty, is adhered to even in gyms and fitness centers. Older men are careful to wear the maximum, often times designer athletic attire when working out.

That sentiment is captured in the admonition, "Clothes make the man." But what happens when a man or woman makes the conscious choice not to wear any clothes. That person regards clothes as not making the man (and woman) but limiting, stifling, and confining them. They see clothes as unnatural to the body. Millions have that view and they are frequently the target of fierce scorn, and equally fierce praise.

Chapter 6

Put Some Clothes On!

The topper among the digs I got for the revealing photos of myself performing asanas in a brief bathing suit came from one Facebook friend. She flatly and very publicly said, "I just couldn't bear to look at those pictures of you naked, so I didn't." If she was shocked at pictures of a man in a bathing suit doing yoga, then she'd probably have to have someone call the paramedics if she happened to click on one of the Facebook groups that have cropped up in recent years that promote yoga in the total buff. One of the nude yoga sites flatly and tantalizing promises that "BOLD & NAKED YOGA employs an explosive blend of athleticism, artistry, power, style and insight to create an experience that makes you feel alive."

This is tame stuff compared to the pictures of the hundreds that mobbed the Palais de Tokyo, a contemporary art museum in Paris for an exhibit it called *visite naturiste* in May 2018. The twist was that all who viewed the exhibit had to do it stark naked. The curators said that they had expected at best a few hundred persons to be interested in the viewing. They were stunned when thousands applied for the very limited number of tickets available. The president of the Paris Naturist Association said that more than two million people visited the group's Facebook page after the exhibit opened. The Paris museum is not unique. There have been other exhibits at museums in other European cities that required that the viewers strip naked. Each time the crush of persons has been overwhelming.

Why would anyone want to look at paintings in the nude? The curators of the exhibit said this engendered a more intimate, and personal feel for the works. In centuries past, the great European art and sculpture masters delighted in erecting dozens of nude sculptures and painting many scenes of frolicking men and women in the buff their great masterpieces. You can't travel through a European city without seeing one of the nude art pieces somewhere.

This was Europe. The liberal, nonchalant attitude of Europeans toward undress, stands in stark contrast to the uproar that a similar exhibit might get in America. That's not speculation. In 2007, a throng of Catholic protesters in New York shut down an exhibit in the city that displayed a completely naked sculpted Jesus. This was too much to bear for those who saw this as blaspheming the image of Christ. The press loved the story. It played it up for all it was worth. Yet, photographers were careful to take pictures, and editors to print, them of the naked Christ's backside only.

When I read that story, I instantly thought of another close friend who after viewing my yoga pictures, gently asked if I had plans to take some more yoga pictures. She said if you do how about this go-round taking the shots in some trendy yoga designed outfits. This was a polite way of saying, please put some clothes on this time.

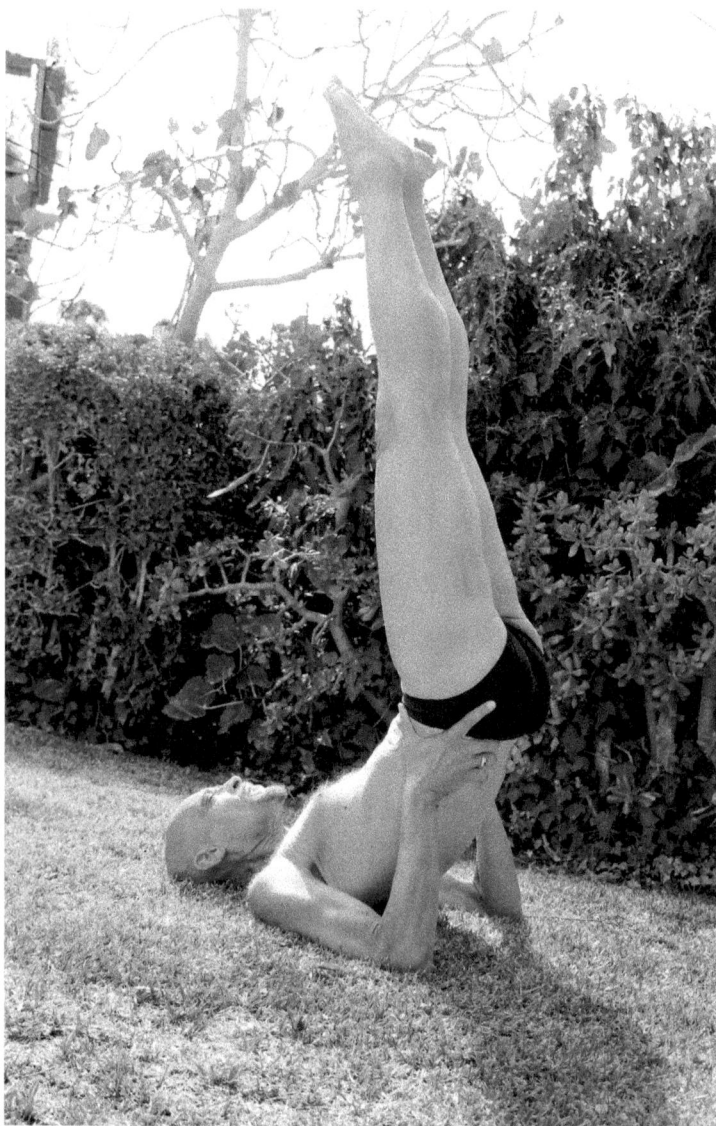

* * * * *

The near hysterical reaction to an older man not nude mind you, but in a bathing suit in Europe would elicit gales of laughter. In the Netherlands public nudity is not only allowed there's even a law that permits it. There are nature societies and federations all over the place in those countries. It's common to see many Europeans tossing off their clothes and working in their gardens and other outdoors places. During a trip to Martinique, my wife and I got in the spirit by stripping off our clothes at one of the nude beaches there.

There are many public places in Europe beyond the old established nude beaches or clothing optional beaches where people routinely romp around naked. The sight of older men parading around naked in these public venues draws not the slightest raised eyebrow. That's not generally the case though in the U.S. where the aversion to nudity still runs deep in wide circles, especially among hard core Christian evangelicals. They almost always dredge out the *Bible* to make their case that parading around naked is an abomination.

No mention is made of the very nude Adam and Eve in *Genesis.*

This aversion toward nudity is, of course, stuffed with hypocrisy. Janet Jackson brought down the wrath of the morals police for her infamous "wardrobe malfunction" at halftime at the Super Bowl in 2004. There was talk of hefty fines for the network and solemn promises from TV industry executives that there would be no repetition of that. They vowed to clean things up. PBS even issued a sort of *mea culpa* about nudity when it put a disclaimer "for mature audiences only" on footage of Michelangelo's very naked sculpture David.

Yet, millions of Americans routinely gawk at the scantily clad Victoria's Secret models that stride across the stage on television and pack the arenas to watch equally scantily clad guys flex their muscles in body building competitions. And while there has been a marked increase in the number of nude beaches in the U.S., there is still a hush hush around them. They are treated as if they are the province of cultists and voyeurs.

* * * * *

Then there's the question of age. That is the perennial phobia of seeing older men and women in a state of undress. Dove soap pulled commercials in 2007 after the FCC banned a series of ads that featured six middle aged women in the nude for Dove Proage products. The FCC would almost certainly have not uttered a muttering word about the ad if the nude women had been 20- year-olds. The conflicted message is that soft porn and mayhem is OK, but nudity will always be frowned on, especially if those nude bodies are older bodies.

The issue roared to the surface again in March 2016, when Kim Kardashian posted a nude selfie. It didn't quite ignite the storm that Jackson's "equipment malfunction" did, mostly because Kardashian has practically feasted off public displays of her body. Kardashian or no, the selfie still raised some eyebrows. However, she had a lot of defenders and they showed their support by posting a rash of their nude selfies. Kardashian actually had the last word on the issue, and it was a good one: "It's 2016. The body-shaming and slut-shaming—it's like, enough is enough. I will not live my life dictated by the issues you have with my sexuality.... I am a mother. I am a wife, a sister, a daughter, an entrepreneur and I am allowed to be sexy."

So, if Kardashian still got a backlash for her nude selfie in 2016, the question is how much has really changed for some Americans when it comes to nudity. Jennifer Jackson had a troubled answer to that. She became the first African-American to pose nude for *Playboy* magazine in March 1965. In an interview in 2011, she confessed that for decades she was so embarrassed and ashamed for posing nude that she didn't tell anyone about her racial breakthrough as the first Black Playboy Playmate in a photo shoot. This changed when she went to a reunion of Playboy Playmates 30 years after her nude shoot.

When she finally got up enough nerve to go public with it, well, here's how she described the reaction, "It was a shock to my sisters because I didn't tell anyone until after I took the picture. And I didn't feel proud of it; I was kind of ashamed of it for a long time." Jackson made it clear that she no longer felt any shame about her nude pose. But the point is it still took her more than 30 years to come to that realization that there was no shame to that.

A reason for the hysteria is the conflicted attitude toward sex in America. It's the stuff of fantasy, lust, and puritanical aversion. Somehow nudity has gotten mixed up in the minds of many with sexual lust and uncontrolled sexual impulses and desires. This brings us back to the picture of an older man, me, in a *Speedo* doing yoga. The beauty of the yoga poses and the mental and physical skill that's required to go through the progression of asanas is totally lost on the viewer who can't get past the undress. Sex is tightly wound up there somewhere, and all that it implies, namely indecency, when a man is not fully dressed.

In the past couple of decades, there's been a slight sea change in how many Americans regard nudity. There are bikeathons in some cities without clothes. They attract hundreds of cyclists. The rub though is that most of the participants are young, and white. So, it's easier not to avert the eyes and chalk that up to young people engaging in a faddist venture, indulgence, or even if there's a sexual spin, to see this as the kind of thing young persons are prone to do.

It would be a far different matter if the participants were older women and men. The verbal darts would fly and there'd be cries to ban such displays of "indecent" public exposure. If the older men and women were of color, it would be pandemonium. There's little chance of that happening. The concept of going bare is just too alien for many older women and men of color. In fact, many of them would lead the charge against such a happening.

When my Facebook friend very pointedly said, "I just can't bear to look at your yoga pictures," I had to at least admire her honesty. She sincerely believed that I had violated the informal social code on what's appropriate when showing the body. I wondered, though, how she'd react to the showcase event in many cities where men and women are attired in less than I was. The showcase event is body building. In recent years, it's attracted a growing number of seniors. They have no reservations about putting their bodies on full display.

Chapter 7

When Body Beautiful is More than a Contest

The body building business is indeed big business in the U.S. There are hundreds of body building showcase events and championship contests held annually in the U.S. Thousands of individuals compete in some cases for big prize money in the various weight, and division categories for the crown of national Body Building Champion. There is one body building event, though, that's a little different. Not that the men and women contestants don't possess fine, muscular chiseled, and rippling svelte physiques. They do. The one slight difference is their age. Many of the contestants are aged 50 plus.

Since its inception a few years back the NPC Southern States Championship held in Fort Lauderdale, Florida has grown by leaps and bounds. The contest now draws hundreds of competitors in the various senior age categories. When they strut across the stage, flexing, primping, and styling for the judges, it's nearly impossible to guess that many of them are 50, 60, or even 70 plus years old. But they are.

Their presence demolished yet another myth, actually two myths. One is that weight training and older age are as incompatible as oil and water. The other is that it's virtually impossible to have a finely toned, muscular body, worthy of putting on display in the barest of bikinis in full public view.

The competitors pretty much all told interviewers the same thing when asked why they do it. It makes them feel great and that by showcasing their bodies, it could motivate other seniors to as one put it, "get on their feet."

In recent years, there's been a rash of articles on the benefits of weight training for seniors. There's a reason. As we age we lose muscle mass. A 60-year-old man, for instance, could lose up to 10 percent of muscle mass. The experts emphasize that working with light weights can improve flexibility, strength, and help minimize the risks of osteoporosis for older men and women. Studies have found that a consistent muscle training program can even reverse some of the effects of muscle loss in the over 60 aged crowd.

Body building and body display for seniors takes this to a whole different level. Here there are similarities with younger body builders and differences that aged 60 plus body builders bring to training and competition. In competition, they still must perfect 8 to 10 poses. They are judged on their grace, muscle symmetry, definition, and body shape. There's also a required choreographed routine to music in many contests.

The difference is that younger body builders want bulk and brawn, and as much of it as they can possibly pack onto their frames. The temptation to cheat for many is often too great. Many have been nailed for the illicit use of steroids and other banned concoctions that promise spectacular muscle gains.

Older body builders pretty much play it straight

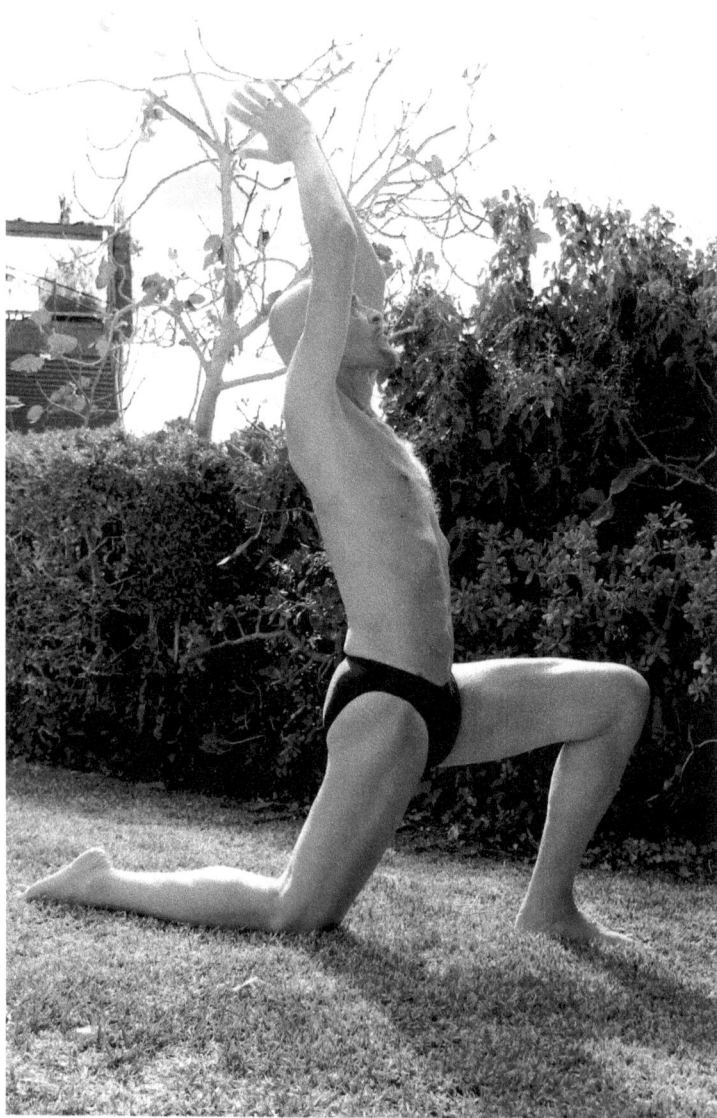

to the vest and only in the rarest of cases have been caught using banned substances. Their goal is different. They want the muscle tone, but that's to improve their physique, not to be top heavy with bulging muscles. This is an important distinction to make. What 60 or 70-year-old man would be delusional enough to think that no matter how good their genes and conditioning, they are going to look, let alone compete with, a 20 or 30-year-old in the body building world?

The motivation and incentive to look the best they possibly can in their clothes and out of their clothes in a skimpy bathing suit is strong. Yet, it generally doesn't cancel out a senior competitor's good sense about their body and age.

For most over aged 60 body builders, just hearing someone say, "You really look good," without the disclaimer, "for your age" is the real pay-off for the time and effort they spent in maintaining and improving their physique. This was certainly true for one competitive bodybuilder who won the Natural Physique Association's Natural Mr. USA bodybuilding championships for men older than 70. He was 77.

"I love to get in front of a crowd, and it is quite a

boost when bodybuilders decades my junior gush: "I'd be so happy if I could look as good as you."

The younger guys did not see him as an aberration but as one of their fraternity of competitive body beautiful enthusiasts.

* * * * *

The Florida competition had 300 seniors compete in the older age group categories in 2015. There were tons of pictures taken of the contestants on stage, off stage, and in the warm-up rooms before each on stage appearance. Their presence got fairly widespread press coverage. However, there was no hint in the coverage that the competitors were somehow just mere curiosity items and that they were in any way different than the younger competitors.

This is important. It's important for the senior body builders who did not see themselves as anything other than serious body builders. And it was important in helping to change the general public's negative perception of older men and women with well-honed muscular physiques, and who had no hang-ups about displaying their physiques in bare bikinis.

Judging from the growing number of testimonials, and on-line articles, and websites by senior body builders, the number of the age 60 plus persons interested in and engaged in weight training program will almost certainly continue to grow. It's a good bet that some of them will even join the ranks of senior body builders and one day find themselves parading across a stage in a showcase body building contest in a tiny bikini.

They may well get the same satisfaction that one senior body builder got before he took up competitive body building, when standing in front of the mirror one day with only his skivvies on, admiring his physique. His son shouted out, "Dad put some clothes on." Months later, and many training sessions later, this champion senior body builder noted with a smile, "I no longer hear that from my son."

Body builders, though, are unique for another reason. There is no shortage of men who compete in that world. It's a far different story for other fitness activities where men are a scarce commodity. Here many who study fitness, health, and wellness issues routinely ask, "Where are the men?"

Chapter 8

Where are
the Men?

After our regular Saturday morning walk and run, my wife and I go to a nearby Starbucks and treat ourselves to tea and a bagel. Along the way we pass two neighborhood fitness centers. There is always a parade of participants leaving the center for a warm up or cool down run or walk. I'm always struck that the workout buffs are almost all women. These aren't aged 20 something women. There is a good mix of 40 plus aged women in the group.

I'm also struck by the looks on their faces as they walk or jog along. They look really determined to make the most of their workout. My guess is that the prime motivation for many of them working out is weight loss. If the weight loss, and the desire to have the body look that gives one pride and self-satisfaction is a powerful motivator, then why don't I see more men among them? It takes work and consistency to attain the benefits, and the women, especially older women, are willing to make the effort. So, again, why aren't more men, especially older men, willing to do the same?

A team of researchers asked that same question. The answers were published in a revealing article in *Psychology Today* in 2013. They noted that in two of the hottest exercise forms, Zumba and Pilates, one would have to search hard to find more than a few men in any of the thousands of these classes nationwide. The answers the men gave ranged from lack of time to the belief that these exercises were strictly for women.

The great irony is that both Pilates and Zumba were created by men. Zumba by a Columbian, Alberto 'Beto' Perez who founded Zumba Fitness in 2001 with two other guys. It is based on Latin dance movements created by Alberto Perlman and Alberto Alghion. Meanwhile, Pilates was founded by a German,

Joseph Pilates, back in the 1920s. The dearth of men in popular exercise programs is even more curious since men dreamed up and organized health and fitness clubs in the U.S. The health fitness boom in the 1960s was made popular by Jack LaLanne. He was hardly a spring chicken. LaLanne sold his fitness program to millions by a shrewd advertising and marketing campaign that featured him flexing his muscular chiseled frame. He looked like an old guy who could still workout with the best of the best athletes. He parlayed it into a multi-million-dollar fitness and health growth industry.

However, the majority of LaLanne enthusiasts weren't men, but women. I still remember my mother sweating and grunting through a series of LaLanne exercises. LaLanne was her lifeline in her battle to shed some unwanted pounds. My father, by contrast, would just look on and grunt and walk on.

* * * * *

Then there's yoga. It's an Eastern world creation, by men. Yet, in America and some European nations, one would have to search hard to find large numbers of men in any of the thousands of yoga classes and workshops held round the clock in America. Even two of the more popular yoga offshoots, hot yoga and Iyengar yoga were created by men.

In my yoga classes at West Los Angeles College most classes average between 25 and 30 students. If there are a half-dozen men in the class, it's a rarity. The only time that the number of men in a class increases is when there's an influx of athletes who need to take the class to satisfy an elective. This further feeds the widely prevalent notion that yoga is a "woman's thing." That notion is reinforced by the fact that most of the instructors are women. I have never had a male yoga instructor in the many years that I have been a yoga practitioner. According to the *Yoga Journal's* 2016 survey, the overwhelming majority of yoga participants in the United States are women. While more men are embracing yoga, they are mostly younger men. I am almost always the only man aged 40 plus in my classes.

Fitness center operators and promoters have long known that women are much more likely to join a fitness center and stay with an exercise program much longer than men. They deliberately tailor their adver-

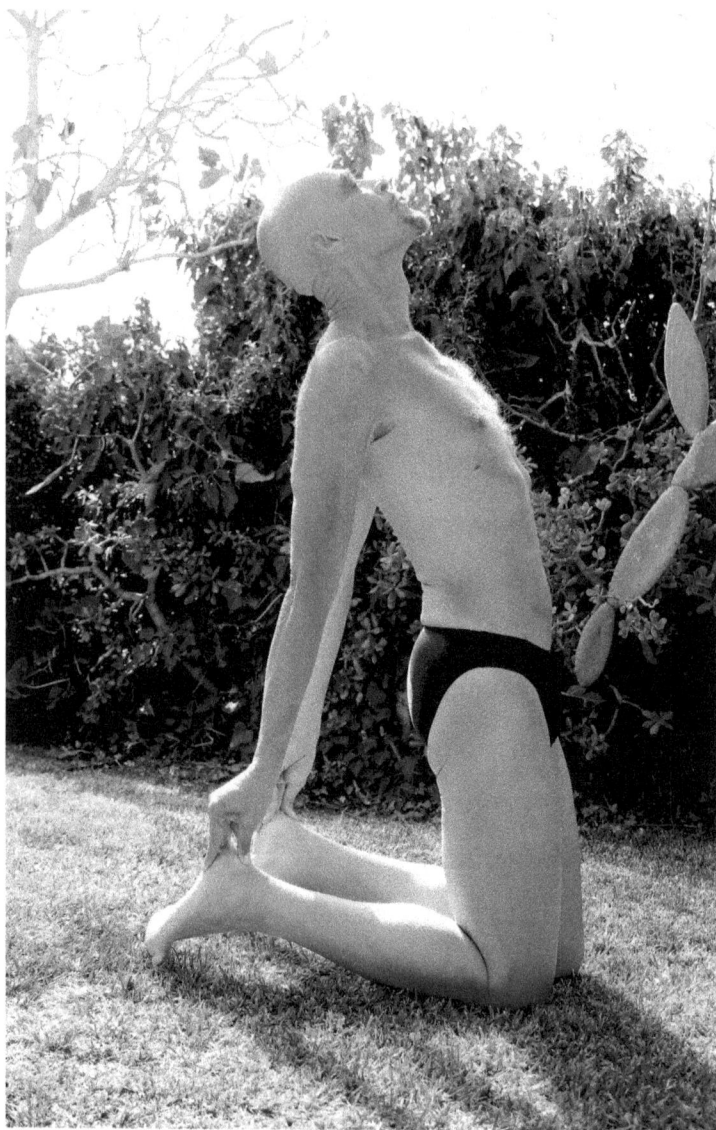

tising pitches to women. More often than not those pitches are to older women. The message to them is they too can be body beautiful and fit just as if they were in their 20s. I have never seen an advertising pitch to older men in any fitness center program.

Older men are not even a bare afterthought. Marketing agencies will not throw their client's dollars at a market that is seen as nonexistent at best, and hostile at worst, to their product. Older men definitely fit that perception when it comes to fitness advertising in the U.S.

The picture is much different in Australia and New Zealand where many of the fitness classes and centers are run by men. A large number of men are in these classes at the centers there. The absence of older men in the centers, and exercise classes and programs is compounded by the age factor.

*   *   *   *   *

Millions of younger men may not do yoga, Zumba, or Pilates, but they do work out, and legions of men work out a lot and consistently. They are in weight training programs, boxing clubs, on the handball and tennis courts. For a lot of them, the goal is to get bigger and stronger, and to look it. That's the embedded male ideal of fitness and good looks. Some of these men, have few qualms about sporting their bodies nude, or in *Speedo* bikini bathing suits. But, for the most part they are aged 20 and 30-year-old guys. There are few aged 50 plus men that fit that bill.

There are varied theories that attempt to explain why that is. They focus almost exclusively on gender. Generally, men are super image conscious of their body. If they don't see themselves as conforming to the male muscular ideal, then forget it. For most older men that image simply doesn't apply. That's especially true for men who participated in high school sports as teens. Many still have pictures of themselves in their high school jerseys or in shorts. They look lean, trim, fit and youthful. As older adults, those days seem light years away from that time in their lives. Few delude themselves that they could get that youthful body look again.

Then why commit to a regular exercise program? For those older men who start on an exercise program, often after they had a health challenge such as a heart issue, or diabetes, and they seek to alleviate the risks, the question then is what kind of exercise program?

Yoga et al. generally aren't the options they choose. Running, biking, and weight lifting also are generally shunned. Usually their workout is a walk, or riding a stationary bike, or a treadmill for a few moments a day, several times a week. This is fine. But will they stick with it? They will if they can see an immediate pay-off. That pay-off is not necessarily getting the obvious health benefit from a dedicated workout regimen. It's how their body will look to them and how others will see their bodies.

This comes full circle back to the idealized fantasy image of what a man's body should look like. Image is a powerful driving force for older men. If I put a lot of work and the flab is still there when I strip down, then the thought is why bother?

Many soon join the millions of other exercise drop-outs. The dismal figures on these fitness drop-outs confirm that a lot of men do join fitness center and programs, but they don't stick with them. In 2015, twenty-five percent of the 41 million health-club members in the United States were over 55-years-old.

Analysts with American Sports Data say this has been the fastest-growing segment of health-club memberships since they began studying fitness gym trends in 1998. They add that the number of active participants who visit the gym at least 100 times per year in the 55-plus category jumped 33 percent, compared to just 13 percent for the under age 34 group. This is misleading. Studies show that nearly half will drop out after a few months.

* * * * *

There are hopeful signs, though, that older men are becoming more dedicated to wellness, and taking a more benign view of their body, even flaunting it. The surge of health and wellness Facebook groups frequently post pictures of aged 50 plus men in shorts, bathing suits, or athletic wear with their chests bare. Many of them have embraced veganism. They look great.

Studies have shown that peer reinforcement is a powerful motivator for older men. That is having more men their age as instructors in fitness programs, and more men their age in these programs. This creates the kind of warm and friendly environment that encourages more older men to participate in and stick with a wellness program.

The sight of older men in shorts and tank tops, no matter what shape their body is in goes a long way toward shattering the stereotype and conception that fitness and displaying one's body is strictly a young man's game. The older men who serve as fitness models for other older men are the men who have answered the question, "Where are the men," with "We are here."

Chapter 9

Getting Past the Yoga is a Girly Thing

In my earlier book, *A Skeptic's Guide to the Yoga Experience,* I wrestled long and hard with myself over rather to add a section in the book on yoga myths, and falsehoods for men over aged 50. One reason I finally decided not to include a section in the book on that was frankly because it was just too close; too close that is to me as an older guy who is deeply involved in the practice.

The other reason was that I didn't think it wise to make age distinctions in yoga. The conventional wisdom and pitch for yoga is that it's a practice that anyone at any age can practice. Talking age, I felt, would just make it seem like there's some kind of stigma for older adults, especially older men, when it came to exploring the benefits of yoga.

Still, the omission of a discussion of age in relation to yoga nagged at me. There were not many over aged 40 participants in my yoga classes at colleges. The ones who were there were almost always women. There are throngs of older women in yoga classes. And this strikes to the heart of the notion held by many that yoga is for women of any age.

That notion has been debunked in numerous articles that tout the benefits of yoga for men of any age. Those benefits are exactly the same as those for women of any age such as increased flexibility, improved muscle tone, and a tension and stress reliever. There is some medical evidence that yoga workouts release the hormone Oxytocin. This has been cutely labeled the "love hormone." It's the hormone that promotes feelings of well-being and happiness. Medical experts say that this reduces anxiety, increases sexual intimacy, as well as the desire for social interaction and lower blood pressure. If yoga is scientifically proven to do any one of these things that in itself should be enough to ignite a stampede by older men to take it up.

For those who want to go deeper with the practice, there's the promise of spiritual awakening and discovery. The physical, mental and spiritual pluses are the very qualities that drew me to yoga, as is true with thousands of others.

The question then is if there are so many possible positives to yoga why aren't older men who are at the greatest risk from almost all of the major health maladies filling up the yoga classes? The easy explanation that it's a "woman's thing" does not totally answer that question. Women have been on the tennis and volleyball courts, the golf courses, and the ice skating rinks, for years. Yet there's no shortage of men in these sports.

* * * * *

One explanation makes more sense. That is that yoga is a kind of mystical, New Age, even gimmicky practice. That's what I thought for years. I just did not see yoga as anything but a slightly mysterious, almost foreign, fad. I certainly did not regard it as an activity that offered any real physical or muscular benefits, let alone mental or spiritual benefits. It took my accidental back-in to the yoga class at a college to strip away the negatives I had long heard and long believed about yoga.

However, even after taking the full plunge and becoming a true believer in it, I still had to fight off the strong urge to find any flimsy excuse to skip the classes. Then it hit me why. It took work, a lot of it, to get some of the intricate poses just right, or some facsimile of them right. It wasn't just the work required. It was boring at times having to go over and over the same moves to get them right. If I felt that way, and I was committed to the practice, it didn't take much to see that for many older men the work and the boredom would be a huge disincentive for them to consider it.

Even the many health benefits that yoga promises to deliver aren't enough for another reason. If I have a back ache, rather than engage in a taxing, possibly demanding yoga workout, why not just get an injection? That doesn't take any work, effort, and it gives instant relief. In America's over medicated, instant gratification, culture, for millions, that, and not yoga, is just what the doctor ordered for pain relief. Despite

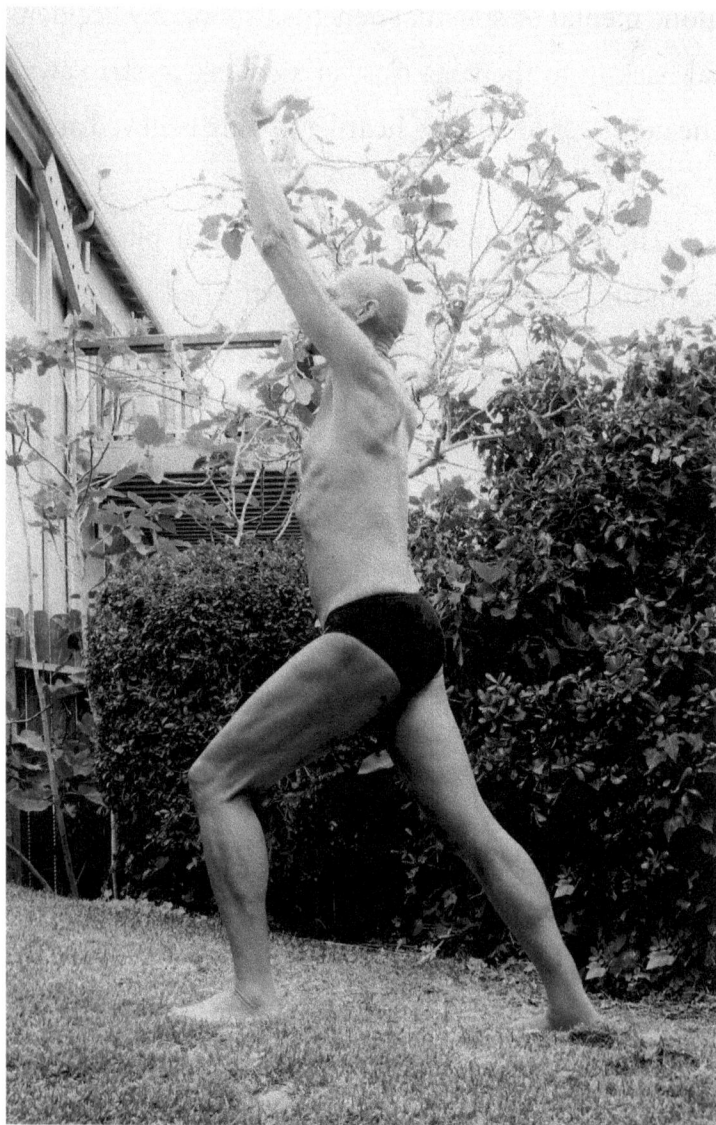

the fact that more doctors are recommending yoga for those various aches and pains to older men, the retort from most of older men is just give me the shot Doc.

There was some hope that the sight of brawny NFL guys doing asanas in the gym and on the football practice field might make yoga seem a palatable workout activity for older men. That happened in 2009, and for a couple of years after. Several NFL teams brought some leading yoga instructors to their training camps. They walked players through some of the yoga positions. The idea was to use yoga to improve flexibility as a means of cutting down the ever-present risk of injury to players in the greatest impact sport, pro football.

There were lots of pictures taken of 300-pound plus linemen doing various poses. There were a spate of articles on the NFLers doing yoga. Though the benefits to the players were constantly played up, it made almost no impression among older men. That definitely included those who bought into the myth that it was too feminine and girly for them. There was no noticeable rush by men to yoga classes.

There were two other glaring reasons for men's reluctance to consider yoga. One, the football guys were young guys. Two, they were athletes. So, anything, including yoga, that could improve their play on the field was seen as simply part of their training, like lifting weights and doing wind sprints, and hitting the tackling dummy. There was little chance that a layman would regard this as anything other than a part of their football training regimen.

* * * * *

There's a few other pet items that some, and I emphasize some, yoga instructors incorporate at the beginning, or during or at the end of their yoga sessions. They chant, go through the Sanskrit words and definitions of the asanas, and play New Age sounds or music. This is OK. The problem though is that these are things that reinforce the feel that yoga is a mystical, counter-culture, New Age, fad. This is a turn-off for many men, and a game killer for most older men.

Chanting, clapping, and lectures in Sanskrit have been rare in the classes I've taken. Soothing music yes, but that's the only departure from getting down to the business of learning and practicing the poses.

The goal is to keep it simple, gentle and relaxed.

This is the key to getting the attention and then participation of men. When the emphasis is on the health benefits of the exercise, it's safe ground for many men that want to give it a try. That's particularly important in most yoga classes where the majority of participants are going to be women.

Another trouble spot is the very thing that gave birth to yoga: spiritualism. This is deeply embedded in the core philosophy of yoga. The heavy emphasis on meditation, concentration and focus, deep breathing, the search for inner peace, and the many preachments about universal belief and faith, are intimate components of yoga thought.

This is hard to stomach for many older men, particularly if they see this as something that sounds New Age, and from an Eastern or Indian religious practice. For a rock-slid Christian evangelical, yoga is something almost akin to the anti-Christ. There have even been some preachers who have railed against it as just that, or at the very least, something that's morally subversive and to be avoided, if not opposed.

* * * * *

It's much safer when trying to sell the benefits of yoga to older men to keep the emphasis on it as a practice to relieve stress and minimize or prevent injury. The injury prevention aspect is especially important because there's enough evidence that men are more injury-prone doing some yoga poses than women. They are bigger, have more bulk, and less elastic muscles, so this is no surprise. This is all the more reason to pitch it as a gentle movement exercise, that can help improve flexibility, and thereby minimize injury. One writer who looked at the gaping disparities between men and women in yoga even flatly said: "You start to get the impression that modern yoga isn't really made for men. It seems like it is designed for women and their bodies and their elasticities."

That's hardly true. However, that impression is so widespread that it's more than enough for most older men to shun it. Fortunately, there are enough doctors, health professionals, sports trainers, and male professional athletes who swear by yoga. They provide a mild counter to this. The likelihood, given the one proven health benefit of yoga, namely increased flexibility, and possibly another, mental calming, is that in future years more men's eyes won't glaze over at the mention of trying a yoga session.

*   *   *   *   *

There's one more thing that might make older men more willing to investigate the possibilities of yoga for their health and to improve their body physique. That's to see and talk with men their age who are into yoga. One of the country's more celebrated yogis might have been a great role model for older men on this score. The 60-year-old entertainment mogul Russell Simmons was the talk of the yoga world and beyond in 2015 when he began spreading the gospel far and wide of its many physical and mental rejuvenating benefits. He opened a popular yoga studio in West Hollywood, California and in New York City.

I had long been an admirer of Simmons; not the music mogul Simmons, but the yoga devotee. He seemed to be embodiment of the older aged 60 plus Black man who had embarked on a similar path that I had and found spiritual, mental, and physical strength through yoga. He was a man who was dedicated to spreading the gospel of that path.

This crashed and maybe burned when he was publicly accused of multiple sexual assaults. I say maybe because Simmons publicly anyway appeared to take full responsibility for his acts. He immediately issued a statement that did not try to sleaze out of the allegation with the usual ploys prominent men use when nailed with a sex charge.

He publicly declared that he would relinquish involvement and operation of his lucrative business interests. Finally, he did something that especially caught my eye and heart. He said that he would seek atonement, healing, and perhaps redemption, from what he and I hold dear, that's yoga. He would do that by converting his studio for yogic science into a nonprofit center of learning and healing.

Simmons provided a template for other men accused of sexual misconduct. This is what I would expect from a guy who truly believes in the spiritual healing power of yoga. He showed by his words and to an extent actions that an older man truly attuned to his mind, body and being is not just about physical strength and body pride but taking responsibility for your life and actions. I credit yoga for that.

This is not a small point since Simmons is one of the group of older men who stand to gain great benefit from yoga, or any other activity that promotes wellness. The group is older Black men. It's overblown to harp on the media fiction that they are endangered. It's not an overstatement to say that health wise, they are at serious risk.

Chapter 10

Breaking Through the Stereotypes

The issue of health, wellness and body image has been a perennial subject of great debate among Black men. These concerns can't be separated from how older Black men are perceived and treated. That has a major impact on how they will perceive and treat each other. One way to understand this is to remember that aged 60 plus Black men were once in their 20s.

Two older men underscored the special perils that confront many older Black men, as with young men, when they told of their harrowing experiences being mistaken for the hired help or pulled over by police while driving and having broken no laws. The two older men were former President Barack Obama and former Attorney General Eric Holder. They told their tales of woe based solely on their color and physical appearance in books and in talks at conferences on racial problems and issues.

Countless studies have found that young Blacks in their 20s and 30s are more likely to be jobless, tossed in jail, join gangs, father children out of wedlock, kill other young Blacks and pillage their communities in far higher numbers than young white or Hispanic men. The assault on the self-image of Blacks doesn't instantly end when a man hits the age 40 mark.

The dangling question that the researchers did not satisfactorily answer is why so many Black men have become at risk in America, and just as important, what can be done to reverse it. Discrimination, racial profiling, failing public schools and broken homes are the easy answers that are routinely fingered to explain the crisis. The slash-and-burn of job training programs and dearth of tax incentives for the working poor have certainly helped fuel the crisis.

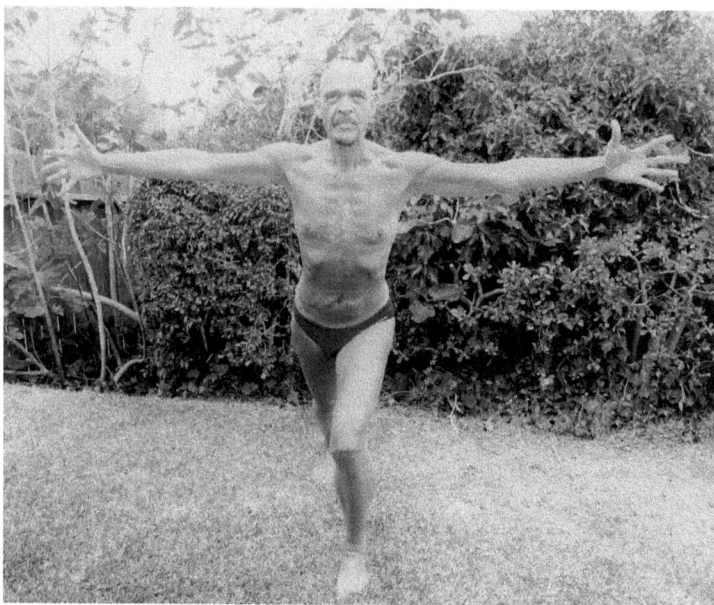

The crisis among Black men can't be solely blamed on dubious fiscal and economic policies. During the Clinton era, when the economy was booming, the unemployment rate for Black males was still double and in some parts of the country triple that of white males. At the same time, state and federal cutbacks in job training and skills programs, the brutal competition for low- and semi-skilled service and retail jobs from immigrants and the refusal of many employers to hire those with criminal records have sledge-hammered black communities. Unfortunately, some Black men reinforce the damaging racial stereotypes by aping and exulting the thuggish bluster and behavior of gangster rappers. This heightens the racially tinged suspicion among some employers that all young Blacks must be criminal and derelict.

This perception holds for older Black men as well. So, the struggle to combat the negative perceptions and typecasting and to come in from the racial cold has taken a predictable turn. That is too tightly embrace and closely conform to the standards and values of American society. There are two perceptions that are especially pernicious and tell much about why many older Black men take an extreme jaundiced stance on anything that steps out of the social norm on wellness and anything other than the most puritanical view of the body.

The first is the perception of Black hypersexuality. It has gotten a lot of Black men killed, jailed, and abused for decades in America. So, the way to counter that is to always try and give the public appearance of being rigid and scrupulous in not saying or doing anything that will further fuel the hypersexual myth. That ties directly into the second way many Black men try to counter the perception of immorality about them.

That is to always be on guard to display in public a prudish and puritan attitude in anything that has even the remotest connection to sex and sexuality, and the display of their body. I made mention earlier that there are hundreds of on-line photos of white guys of all ages, shapes, and sizes, in Speedo briefs, or even less, at beaches, resorts, and doing all kinds of exercise activities. However, I could not find one of a Black man putting their body on like display at any age among the legions of these photos.

* * * * *

This second perception is something that I chuckled at when I published my yoga book not because I found it particularly amusing. The chuckle was to keep from crying at the viciousness of it. The "it" were the homophobic slurs I got from several Black men at my minimally dressed yoga book pictures. This was no surprise. That perception that Black males are hyper-sexually endowed has spurred and intense backlash among many of them to even the faintest hint that they don't fit the conventional notion of what a real man is.

From cradle to grave, the propaganda has been drilled into Black men that the only real men in American society were white men. In a vain attempt to recapture their denied masculinity, many Black men mirrored America's traditional fear and hatred of homosexuality. They swallowed whole the phony and perverse John Wayne definition of manhood, believing that real men talked and acted tough, shed no tears, and never showed their emotions, let alone their bodies, other than in the most macho, exaggerated masculine, rugged guy poses.

These were the prized strengths of manhood.

When men broke the prescribed male code of conduct they were harangued as weaklings, and their manhood questioned.

Many Blacks in an attempt to distance themselves from gays and avoid confronting their own biases dismissed homosexuality as "their thing." Translated: Homosexuality was a perverse contrivance of white males and females that reflected the decadence of white America.

Also, many Blacks listened to countless numbers of Black ministers shout and condemn to fire and brimstone any man who dared think about, yearn for, or engage in the "godless and unnatural act" of having a sexual relationship with another man, or displaying their nude, or scantily clad bodies, to another man.

For many African Americans, Black gay men became their bogeymen and they waged open warfare against them. Black gay men became the pariahs among pariahs, and wherever possible every attempt was made to drum them out of Black life.

Many Blacks tightly embraced traditional religious moral values. This exploded in the great debates in the late 1990s and first decade of 2000 over gay rights and gay marriage. Polls consistently showed that Blacks, especially older Black men, were far more hostile to gay marriage than white males. In time, this slowly changed as gay marriage became legal in more states, and the Supreme Court in a landmark decision in 2015 virtually made it legal nationally.

However, it did not lessen equating masculinity with straight laced heterosexuality. Gay men were still seen as antithetical to Black manhood. This was outrageously evident in the jibes that some Black men took of my photos doing yoga asanas in minimal clothes as "gay stuff."

A close relative aged 60 plus, for instance, just shook his head at the photos. He did not berate me for the pictures, but his visceral reaction of approbation showed that I had somehow stepped way over the line in baring my body. This was just not what men, or maybe a man my age, anyway should be doing. The irony was that he was into yoga. That was of little consequence, since it wasn't the yoga, but my undress that offended him.

The retreat by many older Black men into the traditional values concept of super-masculinity is understandable given the colossal stresses, strains and challenges Black men face. It's not impossible, but it does make it more difficult for many of these men to break out of the patterns and habits of the past. To do that, they'd have to drop their guard and expand their vision to see themselves, and their bodies as well, as something other than a stereotype.

The positive, healthy and gratifying note is the response to my two Facebook groups. One is "Yoga Diversity in Action." The other is "African-American Fitness Past 60." The groups encourage members to post tips, articles, information, ideas and photos on yoga, health, body conditioning. I have posted many of my photos doing varied yoga asanas in the brief. The feedback is always positive from me of all ethnicities. That's a good sign. Some do get it.

Conclusion

A Continuing Wellness Journey

It was a moment in which I felt the world had come crashing down on me in 2010. I just got the word from my primary care physician that I had a pronounced heart arrythmia and that I would have to immediately consult with one of the hospital's cardiologists for further tests. This set off a two-year long series of treatments, intense monitoring, and the insistence that I take one of several recommended heart medications.

The arrythmias got worse and there were more consultations. The recommendation was to have a cardiac ablation. I did. I was warned that the procedure

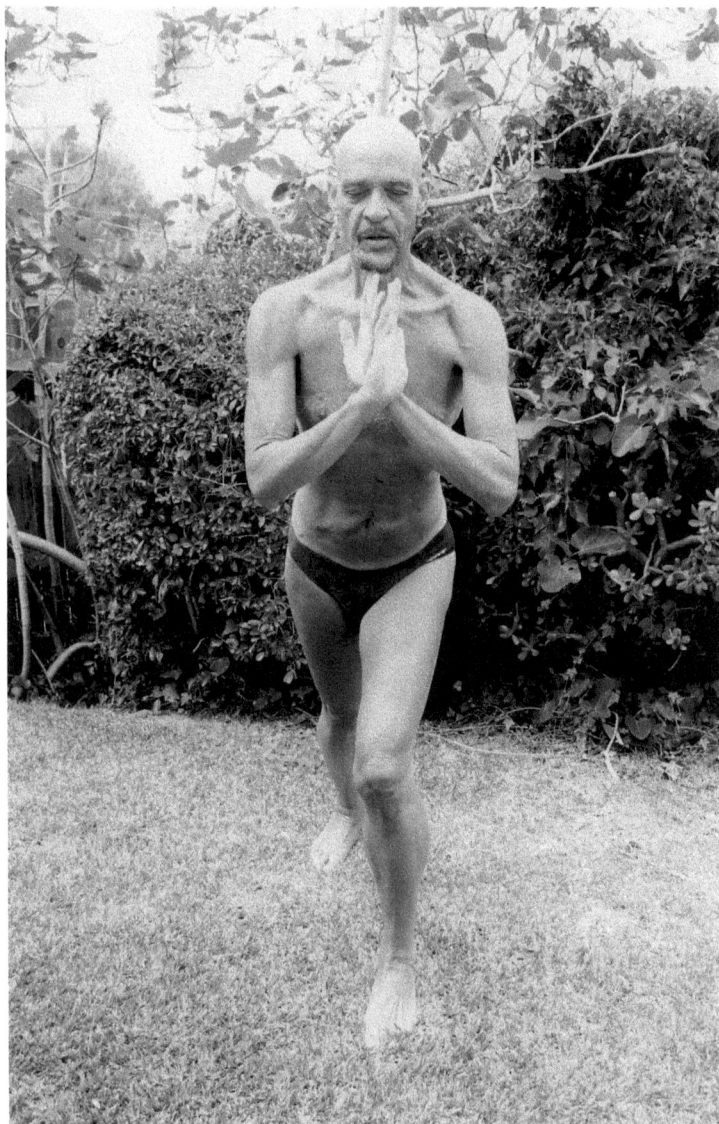

was not fail-safe and that there was a chance that the arrythmias could return. The great danger from them is heart failure and strokes.

Six months later, the arrythmias returned. I had good days and bad days. By far, it had the greatest debilitating effect on me during my almost daily exercise regimen of running, biking, and light weight lifting. This was a regimen that I had maintained for more than 30 years. But during the workouts, I now suffered shortness of breath, dizziness, and nausea. After many more doctor visits and consults, the recommendation was to try yet another procedure, and a more advanced ablation.

I gave it much thought but finally agreed. This time it worked. However, what I and others have noted about the aftermath of a major surgical operation, is the amount of recovery time required for older men. For me, there was remarkably little time down. I knew why? The years of sweat, energy, and time I had put into my workouts paid dividends. I treated my body with dignity, respect, and pride. It returned the favor in getting me back literally on the road running in a relatively short period of time.

This was not the last time I got a positive return from maintaining a consistent exercise program. I had three other procedures for an inflamed appendix, a worn knee, and a colon biopsy. Each time I was able to recover fairly fast.

My fast recoveries even drew raves from my doctors. One was blunt, 'It's rare to find a man your age who is able to get back on his feet the way you did so fast." I certainly did not regard myself as anything special. I did not harbor any illusion that I was somehow different or better than most men my age who face a major medical challenge. Many of them also quickly overcome it and quickly bounce back. They too took pride in, and care of, their bodies. It paid dividends for them when they needed it.

* * * * *

I know all the major hazards that older men, particularly Black men, face, that put them at mortal risk. I applaud the work of organizations such as the 100 Black Men who for years have been prodding, pleading, and cajoling older Black men to get regular checkups, especially the prostate, and to carefully monitor their health. Their health fairs, workshops, and Real Men Cook events are crucial to getting that message to older Black men.

I want to add to that by using myself as an example of an older man who took it a couple of steps further and became a crusader for wellness. I was determined to show by example that an older body does not have to a body hidden, but a body that can be a model of vibrancy and health, and to take pride in showing it.

My journey into the world of wellness consciousness began that day decades ago that I keeled over on the side of a basketball court. It led me decades later to the world of yoga. Like most journeys, mine has had its ups and downs, and setbacks. Yet, I continued to go forward in my wellness journey.

The funny thing is that I never thought that I would chronicle my journey, let alone try to make it a teaching moment for other men and women my age. Two major driving forces further motivated me to do this. One was my concern over the fears and false-hoods about aging. The other was the towering health risks to older men and women. This made it easy for me to decide to share my experiences, and thoughts on

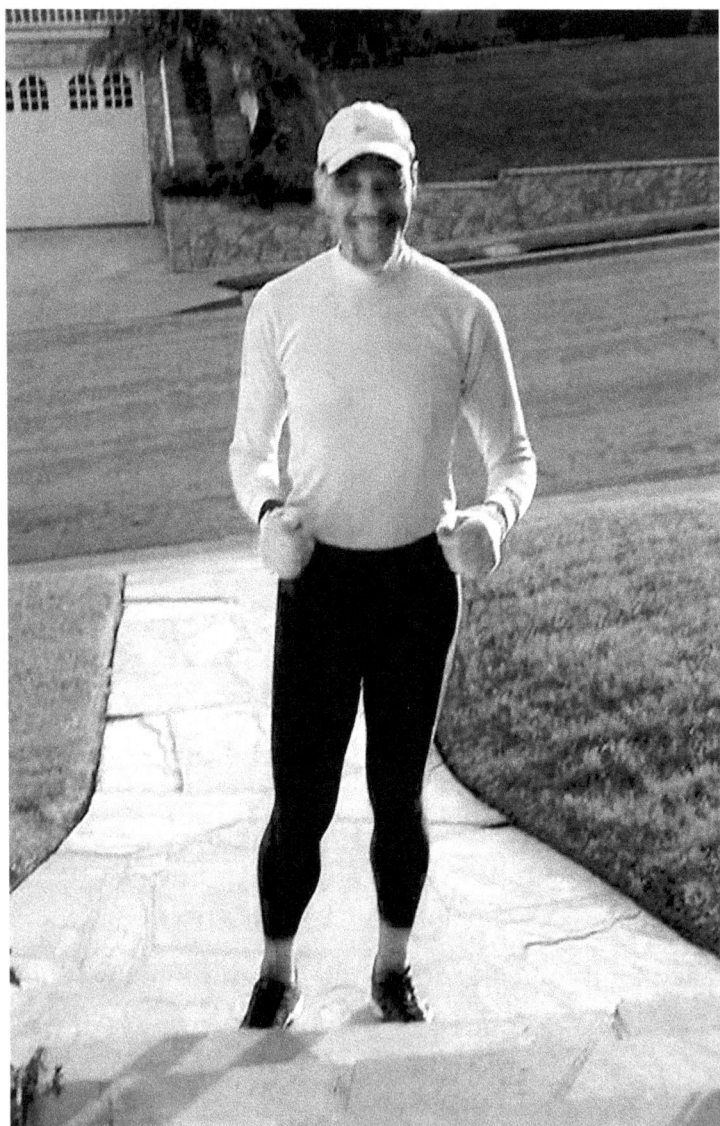

the issue of fitness, wellness, and especially the plague of body shaming. This has done much to inhibit the full blossoming of a massive wellness and body pride movement among older women and men.

* * * * *

In *The Myths of the Asanas: The Ancient Origins of Yoga* by Alanna Kaivalya, she is sometimes called the yoga doctor, she captures the essence of yoga's concept of the warrior. She recounts the story of the two lovers I mentioned earlier who inspired the warrior mythology.

She writes: "Possibly the greatest lesson we can learn from Shiva and Virabhadra is that when we err, we always have the opportunity to step forward and do our best to make things right. Warrior poses are a reminder that ferocity exists not only to destroy but also to allow us sufficient strength to achieve integrity, compassion, and a loving state of mind."

Integrity, compassion, and a loving state of mind are the essence of being a yoga warrior. Despite the snickers and wisecracks from some about my decision to perform yoga asanas in a bathing brief, most loved the pictures and the poses. They understood what I was trying to do. That was to show that an older man could have a body that he took pride in while embracing a spiritual and exercise form that most older men would not consider adopting.

The positive response I got from many to this gave me hope and encouragement. It was this encouragement that further inspired me to write this sequel to my earlier yoga book. A sequel that I hope can serve as an incentive for older women and men to take pride in their body at any age.

Appendix

Three Takes
on Body Pride

Take 1

Body Image Perceptions: Do Gender Differences Exist?

D o men and women experience body image dissatisfaction in the same ways? Do similar factors predict negative body image perceptions in men and women? Is body image dissatisfaction associated with the same consequences regardless of gender? One hundred ninety-seven undergraduate students completed an online survey that assessed their body image experiences and self-perceptions (i.e., body esteem, body mass index, self-esteem, sociocultural and situational factors, and body image perceptions in sexual contexts).

Data analysis compared the responses of male and female participants. Several gender differences were found; body dissatisfaction was more common and felt more strongly in women, yet men were also clearly affected by body dissatisfaction. North American society puts a strong emphasis on physical appearance. People who are deemed attractive are often viewed more favorably than unattractive people. They are thought to be smarter, and more commendable than their less attractive peers. This is also referred to as the "what-is-beautiful-is-good" stereotype.

In our society, attractiveness is associated with being thin for women, whereas a more muscular appearance is considered attractive for men. Appearance ideals are often unattainable for the average person and may be becoming more difficult to meet as the population is becoming heavier. The disparity between "real" and "ideal" size is increasing. How do people respond to this disparity?

It appears that many individuals respond by feeling badly about their bodies and themselves, and subsequently they develop a negative body image. It encompasses an individual's self-perceptions and attitudes about his or her physical appearance. It is useful to view body image as a continuum, ranging from no body image disturbance to extreme body image disturbance.

Another way of conceptualizing how one feels about one's body is called body esteem, which involves an individual's self-evaluation of his or her physical appearance. It has been argued that mass media is a key factor in the development of body image dissatisfaction. The more often an individual is exposed to mass media containing idealistic representations of the body, the less favorable an individual's body image evaluations will become. The mass media influences an individual's perceptions of what the ideal body is, and bodies that do not match this ideal are therefore thought to be unattractive.

Thus, awareness and internalization of society's appearance standards may contribute to body image dissatisfaction. Scrutinizing one's self in comparison to those who are less attractive positively affects self-perceptions. Conversely, comparing oneself to those who are more attractive negatively affects self-perceptions. Therefore, to whom one compares oneself is an important determinant of one's level of body image satisfaction.

Furthermore, believing oneself to be acceptably attractive may be more adaptive than actually being considered attractive by others. How others perceive the individual's attractiveness appears to be less important for an individual's body esteem than how the individual perceives him- or herself.

This suggests that people's perceptions of their appearance are more relevant to how they feel about themselves and their bodies than how closely they actually resemble societal appearance ideals. Lean participants more accurately assessed their body shape than did obese participants, but they were not more satisfied with their appearance. Unfortunately most people experience mild to moderate body image dissatisfaction. People deal with body image dissatisfaction in a wide variety of ways.

A common way of coping is to restrict the number of calories consumed. At any given time, 70% percent of women and 35% of men are dieting. Some individuals resort to extreme forms of caloric intake restriction or develop eating disorders.

Other ways of coping include excessive exercise, cosmetic surgery, and using diet pills, steroids, or protein supplements. Not only does body image dissatisfaction affect one's behaviors, it also affects how one feels about oneself. It is associated with depression, low self-esteem, feelings of shame, body surveillance, diminished quality of life, and anxious self-focus and avoidance of body exposure during sexual activity, which can lead to impaired sexual functioning.

Historically, research on body image dissatisfaction has portrayed it as an issue that exclusively or predominantly affects women. Recent research suggests that the past studies of body image among men were flawed. It was assumed, for example, that body image concerns among men (like those of women) stemmed from perceived excess weight. More recently, studies have been conducted with both men and women using a figure rating scale, where participants rated which figures they actually looked like, wanted to look like, and believed the opposite sex found most attractive.

Men perceived themselves to be more overweight

and more muscular than they actually were. They also believed that the male body women perceived to be the most attractive was significantly more muscular than the actual ideal male body that the women chose.

The research with figure rating scales suggests that men's body image concerns stem from a perceived lack of muscle, whereas women's stem primarily from perceived excess weight. These findings are consistent with media messages that emphasize a thin ideal for women, while promoting a V-shaped figure for men, with emphasis on having a larger, more muscular upper body.

While it is now known that men are also affected by body image dissatisfaction, the literature continues to demonstrate that women suffer from higher rates of discontentment with their bodies and that this discontentment negatively impacts their lives, more so than male body image concerns affect men.

It has been suggested that the ideal male body portrayed in the media is becoming as difficult for typical men to attain as the ideal female body is for typical women to attain. Toys like G.I. Joe are becoming more muscular and, when converted to human size, G.I.

Joe's body is as unattainable for boys as Barbie's body is for girls.

Psi Chi Journal of Undergraduate Research

Fall 2010

http://web.uvic.ca/~lalonde/manuscripts/2010-Body%20Image.pdf

Take 2

Why We Look in the Mirror

We are all more obsessed with our appearance than we like to admit. But this is not an indication of "vanity." Vanity means conceit, excessive pride in one's appearance. Concern about appearance is quite normal and understandable. Attractive people have distinct advantages in our society.

It is not surprising that physical attractiveness is of overwhelming importance to us.

Concern with appearance is not just an aberration of Modern Western culture. Every period of history has had its own standards of what is and is not beautiful, and every contemporary society has its own distinctive concept of the ideal physical attributes. In the 19th Century being beautiful meant wearing a corset—causing breathing and digestive problems. Now we try to diet and exercise ourselves into the fashionable shape—often with even more serious consequences.

But although we resemble our ancestors and other cultures in our concern about appearance, there is a difference in degree of concern. Advances in technology and in particular the rise of the mass media has caused normal concerns about how we look to become obsessions.

How? Three reasons:

1. Thanks to the media, we have become accustomed to extremely rigid and uniform standards of beauty.

2. TV, billboards, magazines, etc. mean that we see 'beautiful people' all the time, more often than members of our own family, making exceptional good looks seem real, normal and attainable.

3. Standards of beauty have in fact become harder and harder to attain, particularly for women. The current media ideal of thinness for women is achievable by less than 5% of the female population.

Even very attractive people may not be looking in the mirror out of "vanity," but out of insecurity. We forget that there are disadvantages to being attractive: attractive people are under much greater pressure to maintain their appearance. Also, studies show that attractive people don't benefit from the 'bias for beauty' in terms of self-esteem. They often don't trust praise of their work or talents, believing positive evaluations to be influenced by their appearance.

IMAGES AND REACTIONS: WHAT WE SEE AND HOW WE FEEL ABOUT IT

What people see and how they react to their reflection in a mirror will vary according to: species, sex, age, ethnic group, sexual orientation, mood, eating disorders, what they've been watching on TV, what magazines they read, whether they're married or single, what kind of childhood they had, whether they take part in sports, what phase of the menstrual cycle they're in, whether they are pregnant, where they've been shopping—and even what they had for lunch.

Sex

All research to date on body image shows that women are much more critical of their appearance than men—much less likely to admire what they see in the mirror. Up to 8 out of 10 women will be dissatisfied with their reflection, and more than half may see a distorted image.

Men looking in the mirror are more likely to be either pleased with what they see or indifferent. Research shows that men generally have a much more positive body-image than women—if anything, they may tend to over-estimate their attractiveness. Some men looking in the mirror may literally not see the flaws in their appearance.

Why are women so much more self-critical than men? Because women are judged on their appearance more than men, and standards of female beauty are considerably higher and more inflexible. Women are continually bombarded with images of the "ideal" face and figure—what Naomi Woolf calls "The Official Body."

Constant exposure to idealized images of female beauty on TV, magazines and billboards makes exceptional good looks seem normal and anything short of perfection seem abnormal and ugly. It has been estimated that young women now see more images of outstandingly beautiful women in one day than our mothers saw throughout their entire adolescence.

Also, most women are trying to achieve the impossible: standards of female beauty have in fact become progressively more unrealistic during the 20th century. In 1917, the physically perfect woman was about 5ft 4in tall and weighed nearly 10 stone. Even 25 years ago, top models and beauty queens weighed only 8% less than the average woman, now they weigh 23% less. The current media ideal for women is achievable by less than 5% of the female population – and that's just in terms of weight and size. If you want the ideal shape, face, etc., it's probably more like 1%.

AGE

Female dissatisfaction with appearance – poor body-image – begins at a very early age. Human infants begin to recognize themselves in mirrors at about two years old. Female humans begin to dislike what they see only a few years later. The latest surveys show very young girls are going on diets because they think they are fat and unattractive. Boys were found to be significantly less critical of their appearance: in one study, normal-weight girls expressed considerably more worries about their looks than obese boys.

Adolescents

Boys do go through a short phase of relative dissatisfaction with their appearance in early adolescence, but the physical changes associated with puberty soon bring them closer to the masculine ideal—i.e., they get taller, broader in the shoulders, more muscular etc.

For girls, however, puberty only makes things worse. The normal physical changes—increase in weight and body fat, particularly on the hips and thighs, take them further from the cultural ideal of unnatural slimness.

Adults

Among women over 18 looking at themselves in

the mirror, research indicates that at least 80% are unhappy with what they see. Many will not even be seeing an accurate reflection.

Research confirms what most of us already know: that the main focus of dissatisfaction for most women looking in the mirror is the size and shape of their bodies, particularly their hips, waists and thighs.

There is some evidence of an increase in body-dissatisfaction among males. As well as some early-adolescent boys, men undergoing the so-called 'male menopause' or mid-life crisis—i.e., men between the ages of about 45 and 55—are most likely to be dissatisfied with their appearance.

When men are dissatisfied, the main focuses of concern are height, stomachs, chests and hair loss. We may see them surreptitiously drawing in their stomachs and walking 'taller' as they pass the mirror.

ETHNIC GROUP

Black and Asian women generally have a more positive body-image than Caucasian women, although this depends on the degree to which they have accepted the beauty standards of the dominant culture.

In a Washington University study, Black women with high self-esteem and a strong sense of racial identity actually rated themselves more attractive than pictures of supposedly 'beautiful' white fashion models. In another study about 40% of moderately and severely overweight Black women rated their figures to be attractive or very attractive. Other research indicates that this may be because African-American women are more flexible in their concepts of beauty than their White counterparts, who express rigid ideals and greater dissatisfaction with their own body-shape.

TV AND MAGAZINES

People's reactions to their reflection in the mirror may depend on recent exposure to idealized images of physical attractiveness. Experiments have shown that people become significantly more dissatisfied with their own appearance after being shown TV ads featuring exceptionally slim and beautiful people. Control groups shown non-appearance-related ads do not change their rating of their own attractiveness.

The same applies to reading fashion magazines. Recent experiments have shown that exposure to magazine photographs of super-thin models produces depression, stress, guilt, shame, insecurity, body-dissatisfaction and increased endorsement of the thin-ideal stereotype.

Mood

Experiments have shown that when people are feeling low or in a bad mood, they experience greater body-dissatisfaction. Most studies have been on women, who also suffer body-image distortion, estimating their size larger, when feeling low.

Childhood

Teasing factor: If you were teased about flaws in your appearance (particularly your size or weight) as a child or teenager, your body image may have become permanently disturbed.

Touch-deprivation factor: People suffering from extreme body-image disturbance report a lack of holding and hugging as children.

Married or Single

Generally, people in stable, long-term relationships have a more positive body-image than singles. This applies to all ages, although an American study of adolescent "dating-behaviour" showed that teenagers who "date" in groups have a significantly better body-image than those go out alone with their boyfriend or girlfriend.

Eating Disorders

Anorexics and bulimics suffer from greater body-dissatisfaction and greater body-image disturbance than other women: these women are even more likely to be unhappy with their reflection in the mirror, and even more likely to see a distorted image.

Sport

Perhaps surprisingly, given that their physique is closest to the stereotype masculine ideal, male body-builders experience greater dissatisfaction with their appearance than almost any other males. Body-builders are generally regarded as vain: in fact they suffer from low self-esteem combined with high perfectionism.

One American study indicates that female body-builders, by contrast, seem to have a more positive body-image than other women. A London University study appears to confirm this, finding that women who take part in sport (body-builders, rowers and net-ballers) have more positive perceptions of their own bodies and increased acceptance of muscular body shapes, despite their divergence from cultural ideals.

It is interesting to note that another study showed exercise therapy to be as effective as conventional psychotherapy in treating serious body-image disturbance in young women. Generally, both men and women who participate in sport have a more positive body-image than those who do not.

Obesity

Fat-phobia and prejudice against the overweight in our culture is such that obese people (particularly women) tend to have a very poor body-image—not to mention severe anxiety and depression (studies have shown the mental well-being of obese women to be worse than that of the chronically ill or even severely disabled). These problems are not caused by obesity itself—in cultures without fat-phobia or where fat is

admired, obese people show no signs of these effects—
but by social pressure and the association of beauty
with thinness.

Social Issues Research Center, London
http://www.sirc.org/publik/mirror.html

Take 3

Naked Yoga Is Here

I n 2013 New York City's Le Male Yoga, which has been offering all-male naked yoga classes in Chelsea for more than seven years, announced it was turning over a new leaf. (And not the kind that covers that area.)

The studio is now called Bold & Naked Yoga and will offer a full schedule of no-clothes classes in 2014, including men's, women's, and co-ed. And lest you imagine an in-person, more to-the-point version of Tinder, the duo says that doing sun salutations in the buff next to other sweaty naked strangers has tons of benefits, none of which are hooking up—like building your confidence, boosting your sex life…and leaving more dough in your bank account for body scrubs.

"The first thing that comes to mind is you save a lot of money—you don't have to spend hundreds of dollars on Lululemon," jokes Joschi Schwarz, who owns the studio with partner Monika Werner. "We are both European, so we are pretty liberal to begin with. I was a little bit scared [of New Yorker's reactions], but New York is coming with us. I hope they will realize how cool and freeing and liberating it can really be."

Will they? We caught up with the duo to find out more:

You've been teaching all-male naked classes for so long. What prompted this expansion?

Schwarz: I'm teaching for over 20 years, and my interest was always in how can I take a subject and translate this into the now, and I mean really into the now, and not just use some kind of quotes and sayings you hear in a regular yoga class that they read from a piece of paper. There are things which are maybe interesting to know and to hear but they can not take this and put this into their daily life. Real life spirituality is the concept. Real. Life. Spirituality. So you walk out and go to your meeting or home to your relationship or whatever the circumstances, and you're inspired to handle the situation a little better and think a little bit differently about it.

Okay, I get the idea, but how does group naked-ness lead to that kind of real life spirituality?

Schwarz: I think social connection, respect, trust, all of these things are very important. And it starts with every individual in class. Being naked has a few factors, and one is to get more confidence and to learn to trust yourself, other people, and the situations and circumstances you're in.

You sit naked in the class and create confidence, and then you go to your next meeting, and of course you're not naked in the next meeting, but you go with more confidence, that's a given. You get to know your-self a little better, and it just goes into all of the situa-tions. That's just one of those big things. Why not start with yourself?

So far you've only taught classes that were all men. Are you sure women's classes, and especially the co-ed version, will work?

Schwarz: I can't talk about co-ed classes yet, but I

think my personality is strong enough that I can lead it. Werner: For women's classes, I think the most important thing is that nudity is still an issue and a social taboo, and we want to work against that because there's nothing more natural than being in the nude.

Women get held to such high standards about what they look like by magazines and Photoshopped images, and to sit and see that everybody has some issues with their bodies and be okay with it—it'll create positive body image. With clothes, you can hide, and when you're naked, you can let it all out. And just to have a group of women together that support each other and to not care about what other people think. When you have more confidence in a naked body, you have more confidence in your clothed body.

Alright, I get distracted when the person next to me coughs or breathes weird in yoga. Isn't it hard to get centered when your neighbor's bare butt is in your face or your own parts are dangling every which way?

Schwarz: Once you start being in the class, the teachers, us, we're professionals, and we create this atmosphere where you feel safe and secure, and once you start moving, your mind comes to the mat. The reality is when you're on the mat, you're on the mat... And guys, if you get a hard-on, and that's just what's happening with your body. I would say just be happy that your reproductive system works. It won't last forever. You won't see a man with an erection going throughout the whole class, though, it's physically not possible.

Um, good to know. On that note, how do make sure there aren't creeps coming just to be creepy?

Schwarz: I know people will come just out of curiosity, so the first class costs more. We want to achieve that there are not people just coming here to see naked people. We have people go a few times to get the feeling for it and the idea of what the whole thing is about.

It's true: they require potential clients fill out a questionnaire before they sign up for a class and offer a co-ed beginner series "Naked Yoga & Tea" for newbies to get comfy with each other. For that visual, I say, you're welcome.

https://www.wellandgood.com/good-sweat/new-bold-naked-yoga-studio-new-york/

Notes

CHAPTER 2
YOU CAN BE A WARRIOR
AT ANY AGE

http://absoluteyogacrosby.co.uk/story-behind-virabhadrasana-ii-iii

www.doyouyoga.com/the-physical-mental-and-emotional-benefits-of-the-warrior-poses/

www.slate.com/articles/business/the_dismal_science/2009/11/are_men_more_competitive_than_women.html

www.unm.edu/~lkravitz/Article%20folder/ExerciseMot.pdf

CHAPTER 3
HEY, YOU'RE TO OLD FOR THAT

www.loudounsportstherapy.com/1294-five-
myths-about-exercising-and-aging

www.cleveland.com/national-senior-games/in-
dex.ssf/2013/07/national_senior_games_oblitera.html

http://aginginstride.enewsworks.com/en/10022/
articles/915/Five-Myths-About-Exercise-and-
Healthy-Aging.htm

www.abcnews.go.com/US/100-year-man-breaks-
world-records-track-field/story?id=33950048

CHAPTER 4
SAYING 'NO' TO BODY SHAMING

www.people.com/bodies/serena-williams-
calls-out-haters-on-instagram/

www.huffingtonpost.com/entry/serena-williams
-sportsperson-year-ceremony-speech_us_5671723
5e4b0dfd4bcbffcbf

www.biblicalgenderroles.com/2015/03/13/why-
nudity-is-not-always-shameful-for-a-christian/

www.consumerhealthdigest.com/female-sexual-

health/8-types-of-sex-that-bring-two-people-closer-
together.html

www.bradley.edu/sites/bodyproject/male-body-
image-m-vs-f/

www.washingtonpost.com/news/morning-mix/
wp/2017/03/14/psychologists-we-see-black-men-as-
larger-and-stronger-than-white-men-even-when-
theyre-not/?utm_term=.8e70e6d8fdac

Chapter 5
Saying 'Yes' to Body Pride

https://ftw.usatoday.com/2017/08/kobe-bryant-
deleted-shirtless-mambathick-photo-instagram-lak-
ers-nba

www.bradley.edu/sites/bodyproject/male-body-
image-m-vs-f/

www.washingtonpost.com/news/morning-mix/
wp/2017/03/14/psychologists-we-see-black-men-as-
larger-and-stronger-than-white-men-even-when-
theyre-not/?utm_term=.8e70e6d8fdac

CHAPTER 6
PUT SOME CLOTHES ON!

www.boldnaked.com

www.nytimes.com/2018/05/07/arts/naked-museum-france.html

www.wbur.org/hereandnow/2016/03/11/debate-over-nude-selfies

www.newsweek.com/hugh-hefner-playboy-african-american-models-673286

CHAPTER 7
WHEN BODY BEAUTIFUL IS MORE
THAN A CONTEST

www.dailymail.co.uk/news/article-2363887/Rise-fit-50s-body-building-competitions-open-categories-senior-citizens.html

www.npr.org/2011/02/21/133776800/seniors-can-still-bulk-up-on-muscle-by-pressing-iron

www.nytimes.com/2008/04/03/fashion/03Fitness.html

Chapter 8
Where are the Men?

www.psychologytoday.com/us/blog/fit-femininity/201308/there-are-no-men-in-my-exercise-class

www.prnewswire.com/news-releases/2016-yoga-in-america-study-conducted-by-yoga-journal-and-yoga-alliance-reveals-growth-and-benefits-of-the-practice-300203418.html

http://cwis.usc.edu/student-affairs/glbss/PDFS/BlackMenMasculinity.pdf

www.qrd.org/qrd/www/culture/black/articles/ofari2.html

http://smallbusiness.chron.com/target-market-fitness-gyms-3354.html

Chapter 9
Getting Past the Yoga is a Girly Thing

www.huffingtonpost.com/rachael-yahne/men-yoga_b_7655114.html

http://health.heraldtribune.com/2013/11/05/why-dont-real-men-do-yoga/

www.newsfeed.time.com/2010/09/22/is-yoga-an-anti-christian-practice/

www.nytimes.com/2012/01/08/magazine/how-yoga-can-wreck-your-body.html

www.hollywoodreporter.com/news/writer-jenny-lumet-russell-simmons-sexually-violated-me-guest-column-1062934

Chapter 10
Breaking Through the Stereotypes

www.thehill.com/homenews/news/215627-holder-tells-ferguson-students-he-was-a-victim-of-racial-profiling

www.huffingtonpost.com/2014/12/17/obama-people-interview_n_6339972.html

www.nytimes.com/interactive/2018/03/19/upshot/race-class-white-and-black-men.html

www.npr.org/templates/story/story.php?storyId=10057104

www.hotair.com/archives/2015/06/08/holdouts-blacks-oppose-gay-marriage-4151-in-new-pew-poll/

www.verywellhealth.com/black-american-mens-health-2328772/

Bibliography

Alsenas, Linas, *Gay America: Struggle for Equality*, New York: Amulet Books, 2008

Anderson, Howard, *Why Nude?: Thoughts and reflections on social nudity*, Copenhagen, Denmark: Naktiv, 2016

Atkinson, Debra, *You Still Got It, Girl! The After 50 Fitness Formula for Women*, Monterey, California: Healthy Learning Publishers, 2015

Bjorn, Nicholas, *Fitness Nutrition: The Ultimate Fitness Guide: Health, Fitness, Nutrition and Muscle Building—Lose Weight and Build Lean Muscle*, Charleston, S.C.: Create Space, 2015

Books, DP, *Nude Yoga: For Body, Mind & Spirit*, New York: DP Books, 2018

Brown, Brene, *I Thought It Was Just Me (but it isn't): Making the Journey from What Will People Think?* *to I Am Enough,* New York, Gotham, 2007

Brown, Harriet, *Body of Truth: How Science, History, and Culture Drive Our Obsession with Weight—and What We Can Do about It,* New York: Da Capo Lifelong Books, 2015

Brown, Christina, *The Yoga Bible,* Walking Stick, 2003

Cole, Campbell, *Yoga: Yoga For Men: Become A Mindful Warrior. Core Strength, Flexibility, Mindfulness,* Charleston, S.C., CreateSpace, 2015

Farrell, Amy Erdman, *Fat Shame: Stigma and the Fat Body in American Culture,* New York: NYU Press, 2011

Galloway, Jeff, *Running Until You're 100,* New York: Meyer & Meyer, 2010

Grufferman, Barbara Hannah, *Love Your Age: The Small-Step Solution to a Better, Longer, Happier Life,* New York: National Geographic, 2018

Hutchinson, Earl Ofari, *A Skeptic's Guide to the Yoga Experience,* Los Angeles: Middle Passage Press, 2017

Jenkins, Jo Ann *Disrupt Aging: A Bold New Path to Living Your Best Life at Every Age,* New York: Public Affairs, 2018

Moffat, Frank T and Roach, Michael T., *Your Second Fifty Rising Above the Myths of Aging,* Victoria, Canada: YSF Publishing, Inc., 2015

Rae, Augustine, *The Freedom of Naturism: A Guide for the How and Why of Adopting a Naturist Lifestyle,* Charleston, S.C.: CreateSpace, 2015

Simmons, Russell, *The Happy Vegan: A Guide to Living a Long, Healthy, and Successful Life,* New York: Avery, 2015

Tarkeshi, Jasmine, *Yoga Body and Mind Handbook: Easy Poses, Guided Meditations, Perfect Peace Wherever You Are,* Sonoma Press, 2017

Taylor, Michael, *Shattering Black Male Stereotypes: Eradicating The 10 Most Destructive Media Generated Illusions About Black Men,* Houston: Creation Publishing Group, 2017

Thelos, Philo, *Divine Sex: Liberating Sex from Religious Tradition,* Bloomington, Indiana: Trafford Publishing, 2006

Vigil, Juan, *Seniors on the Run: Extending Your*

Life One Step at a Time, Charleston S.C.: CreateSpace, 2016

Wescott, Wayne, *Strength Training Past 50,* Champaign, Ill.: Human Kinetics, 2015

Index

About the Author

Earl Ofari Hutchinson is an author of multiple books on race and politics in America. His latest books are How Obama Won and *50 Years Later: Why the Murder of Dr. King Still Hurts* (Middle Passage Press). He is a frequent commentator on *RT America* news and past commentator on MSNBC and CNN. He is a weekly co-host of the *Al Sharpton Show* on Radio One. He is the host of the weekly *Hutchinson Report* on KPFK 90.7 FM Los Angeles and the Pacifica Network.